Living Without magazine's

Best Gluten-Free Cookbook

150+ Allergy-Friendly Recipes From Our Favorite Chefs

Recipes by   Mary Capone   Beth Hillson   Matthew Kadey   Diane Kittle
Robert Landolphi   Rebecca Reilly   Jules Shepard   Sueson Vess

ISBN: 1-879620-97-9

BELVOIR MEDIA GROUP, LLC

800 CONNECTICUT AVE

NORWALK, CT 06854

BOOK DESIGN & FRONT COVER PHOTOGRAPHY BY OKSANA CHARLA

LIVING WITHOUT®

EDITOR-IN-CHIEF **Alicia Woodward, LCSW**
DESIGN DIRECTOR **Oksana Charla**
ASSOCIATE EDITOR **Eve Becker**
FOOD EDITOR **Beth Hillson**
TEST KITCHEN **Madalene Rhyand**
SPECIAL PROJECTS **Laurel Greene**

This book is dedicated to those with
special dietary needs, all who desire to
live well, living without.

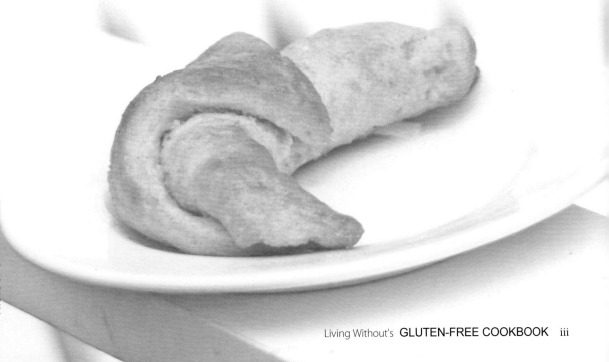

CONTENTS

Contents

Chapter 3: Breads

Chapter 4: Soups

Chapter 5: Main Course

Chapter 8: Bars, Cookies and More

Introduction

Today nearly 20 million people have given up gluten because they have celiac disease or gluten sensitivity—but no one wants to give up pizza, bread, cake and all the wonderful foods of the past. Fortunately, there's no need to give up anything . . . except the gluten.

When readers contact us at *Living Without* magazine, they are often feeling overwhelmed and longing for the foods they think they'll never have again. As we sort through their concerns, we always tell them to look at what they *can* have, not what they've left behind. Then we make a list of all the safe ingredients and add those to their toolbox. Before you know it, they are baking their way back to good health and good food. (These can be one and the same, as evidenced by the recipes in this book.) We can almost sense the happiness returning once people roll up their sleeves and begin to bake.

I've been there. I was diagnosed with celiac disease 35 years ago when there were no resources or prepared gluten-free foods. I went to culinary school to understand recipes and discovered that nearly every baking formula can be made over by replacing regular flour with gluten-free flour. The key is to maintain the original ratio of ingredients and to use excellent substitutions. Substitution is our mantra at *Living Without*, the nation's leading food, health and lifestyle magazine for those with food allergies and sensitivities. We hope *Best Gluten-Free Recipes* helps make it your mantra, too.

This cookbook features eight of *Living Without's* favorite friends—gluten-free chefs, many of them cookbook authors, who work regularly with the magazine. Each of these experts shares our food philosophy:

- Start with an excellent flour blend.
- Use the freshest ingredients for the most vibrant flavors.
- Love nutritionally dense ingredients and they will love you back.
- Keep trying!

At *Living Without*, we welcome each new gluten-free, dairy-free cookbook as we would welcome an honored guest. Each time one is published, it feels like we make a new friend. The author and his or her recipes become part of the special-diet community, enriching and enhancing us all.

We hope you'll welcome this cookbook in the same way and that our chefs will inspire your gluten-free, dairy-free cooking. Perhaps you'll discover a new way of using alternative ingredients, an essential tip about gluten-free flour, a word of encouragement. Maybe one of our chefs will start you on your own culinary adventure.

Whatever you embrace from these pages, make it your own. Let *Living Without's* special-diet expert chefs become your friends and let their recipes nurture your soul.

Beth Hillson
Food Editor
Living Without magazine

About This Book

Welcome to the delicious world of gluten-free, allergy-friendly eating. This cookbook was created to keep you safe and satisfied (deliciously satiated!) on your special diet.

The front section of each chapter features the favorite recipes of one of *Living Without's* celebrity chefs. The back pages contain a collection of winning recipes created by our other expert chefs. Together, these chapters provide delicious recipes for every meal of the day, from appetizers to dessert. Every recipe is gluten-free and we provide substitutions for dairy, nuts, soy, peanuts and often for eggs (if the recipe permits).

Note that a Shopping List of these substitutions, as well as hard-to-find gluten-free or allergy-friendly products, is located on page 189. This is a great guide for preparing these recipes and for stocking your gluten-free kitchen.

Gluten-Free Flour Blends

Gluten is the protein in wheat (barley and rye, too) which delivers structure and elasticity to baked items. When gluten is omitted from a recipe, the end product can be hard and crumbly unless the right alternative is used.

One size does not fit all when it comes to recreating the taste and texture of wheat flour. In gluten-free baking, it's best to use a combination of flours instead of just one type. This is why gluten-free bakers combine different flours and starches to make a flour blend.

Living Without's celebrity chefs use their own signature blends throughout this cookbook. These customized blends help control the outcome and give the baker the best results.

It isn't absolutely necessary to use these customized blends to make the recipes in this book. You can usually use any all-purpose blend from these pages, make your own blend (page xiv) or substitute your favorite commercial all-purpose blend (cup for cup) and usually achieve good results.

Dee's Flour Blend #1
MAKES 3 CUPS
2 cups rice flour (finely ground brown rice flour is best)
⅔ cup potato starch (not potato flour)
⅓ cup tapioca starch/flour

Combine all ingredients.

Dee's Flour Blend #2
MAKES ABOUT 4 CUPS
1⅓ cups brown rice flour (finely ground is best)
1⅓ cups tapioca starch/flour
1⅓ cups cornstarch
1 tablespoon potato flour (not potato starch)

Combine all ingredients.

Dee's Flour Blend #3
MAKES ABOUT 4½ CUPS
1½ cups rice flour (finely ground brown rice flour is best)
1½ cups tapioca starch/flour
1½ cups corn starch or potato starch (not potato flour)
3 tablespoons potato flour (not starch)

Combine all ingredients.

Dee's Pastry Flour Blend
MAKES 3 CUPS
2 cups finely ground brown rice flour
¾ cup potato starch (not potato flour)
¼ cup tapioca starch/flour

Combine all ingredients.

Flour Blends

Living Without's All-Purpose Flour Blend

MAKES 4 CUPS

2 cups rice flour (a combination of white
and brown rice flour works well)
1 cup tapioca starch/flour
1 cup cornstarch or potato starch

Combine all ingredients.

Living Without's High-Protein Flour Blend

MAKES 4¼ CUPS

1¼ cups bean flour (of choice),
chickpea flour or soy flour
1 cup white or brown rice flour
1 cup arrowroot starch, cornstarch or
potato starch (not potato flour)
1 cup tapioca starch/flour

Combine all ingredients.

Mary's All-Purpose Flour Blend

MAKES 6 CUPS

2 cups brown rice flour
2 cups white rice flour
1⅓ cups potato starch (not
potato flour)
⅔ cup tapioca starch/flour

Combine all ingredients.

Making Your Own Blend If you want to make your own all-purpose blend, start with an easy combination of 40 percent rice flour, 30 percent tapioca starch/flour and 30 percent potato starch (not potato flour) or cornstarch. If you prefer a more refined blend, experiment with gluten-free whole-grain flours, like amaranth, sorghum, millet, quinoa, gluten-free oat flour, chickpea flour or buckwheat flour. A good rule of thumb is to use less than 30 percent of one of these high-protein flours in a blend.

It's important to understand the nuances of gluten-free flours and to know which ones give you the best outcome for the type of baked good you're preparing. For instance, amaranth, quinoa, millet, chickpea and gluten-free oat flour are rich in nutrients and high in protein. They add elasticity to yeast breads and pizza—but each has a distinct taste. They aren't recommended in recipes for delicate cookies and layer cakes. For

Flour Blends

these, use rice flour instead, which is more neutral in flavor but contains little protein. In yeast breads, use high-protein flours for the best texture and maximum rise.

Adding Gums Xanthan gum, guar gum and agar powder are heavy lifters in gluten-free baking. They add back some of the elasticity that is missing in gluten-free flours. They also keep the dough moist, as well as add structure and texture.

A little gum goes a long way. Use ½ teaspoon of gum per cup of flour blend for pastries. Use 1 teaspoon of gum per cup of flour blend for yeast dough, such as bread, pizza and rolls.

Substituting a Commercial Blend If you don't have time to make these blends or don't have the ingredients, use a commercial all-purpose gluten-free flour blend. For best results with yeast items, select a blend that contains a high-protein flour, such as chickpea or sorghum.

Read the ingredient list before selecting a blend. Some contain additional ingredients, like powdered milk, almond meal, gelatin or Expandex, which can affect the success of the recipes in this book. Some experimenting may be needed.

In addition, some commercial blends contain xanthan or guar gum and salt. If so, don't add them again when the recipe calls for gum and salt.

If your commercial blend contains only flours and starches, use it cup-for-cup as you would the blend called for in the recipe. Add xanthan gum and salt as directed by the recipe.

Storing Flours Keep gluten-free flour in a tightly covered container in your refrigerator or freezer to extend its shelf life. This is especially important for high-protein flours, flax meal and nut flours.

Baking Tips

House Rules

Read the recipe from start to finish before preparing the dish. Make sure you have all ingredients before beginning.

For best outcome, have all ingredients at room temperature before starting a recipe. The exception is butter or non-dairy alternative. Follow the recipe instructions; it may specify *cold, softened to room temperature, or melted.*

Don't rush. Allow extra time the first time you make a recipe.

Measuring

Dry Ingredients. Use a set of graduated measuring cups that are flat on top to measure dry ingredients. Spoon the ingredient into the cup and level it off with the flat side of a knife or spatula. Do not pack the ingredient into the cup unless the recipe calls for that, such as packed or lightly packed brown sugar.

Liquid Ingredients. Use glass or plastic pitcher-style measuring cups for liquids. Set the measuring cup on a counter and get down to eye level to line up the liquid with the appropriate measuring mark on the cup.

Scoops. Ice cream scoops of varying sizes are perfect for delivering just the right amount of dough for cookies, muffins and rolls.

Instant-Read Thermometer. Purchase an inexpensive instant-read thermometer to check the temperature of warm liquids for yeast bread recipes and the internal temperature of baked bread.

Baking Times

Baking times vary depending on oven and pan size. Begin checking for doneness a couple of minutes before the timer goes off.

Unless your recipe instructs otherwise, cool baked goods in the pan for 10 minutes before turning them onto a wire rack to finish cooling.

Cool cakes and cupcakes completely before frosting.

Dairy-Free

Dairy products add fat, protein and calcium to baked items. Fortunately, there are many dairy-free alternatives on the market. All recipes in this book can be prepared without dairy-containing ingredients. Notations for

Baking Tips

non-dairy alternatives are listed in the recipe ingredients. For a complete list of dairy substitutions, see Substitution Solutions on page 187.

NOTE When used in recipes for baked goods, butter spreads more than non-dairy alternatives. Keep this in mind when making cookies. If your cookies spread too much, reduce the amount of real butter by 2 table-spoons the next time you prepare the recipe or use half butter and half organic shortening.

Egg-Free

Eggs add liquid, fat and protein to bakery items. They act as a binder and help leaven, which affects the texture and density of baked goods. A majority of recipes in this book can be made with egg replacements. We provide instructions on how to do this with the recipe. If a recipe does not work with an egg substitute, we tell you that in the introduction to the recipe. For more about egg substitutes, see Substitution Solutions on page 187.

NOTE Baked goods that use egg replacers will not have the same loft as those produced using eggs. The end result can be a bit more dense and may be somewhat drier in texture. The taste, however, will be comparable.

Yum.

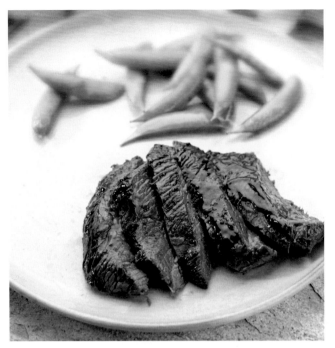

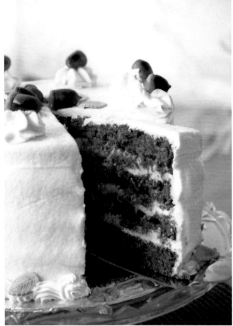

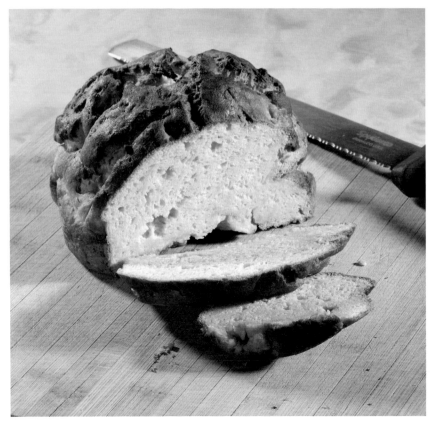

TOP LEFT
Spiced Steak with
Island Barbecue Sauce,
page 117

TOP RIGHT
Apple Spice Cake,
page 160

BOTTOM
Hawaiian Sweet Bread,
page 66

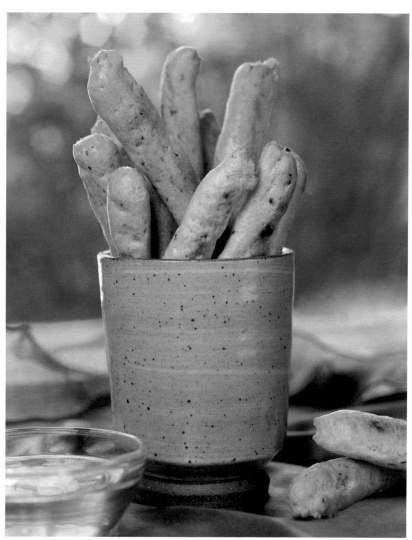

TOP Herb and Garlic
Breadsticks, page 67

BOTTOM Airy Pancakes
with Blueberries, page 12

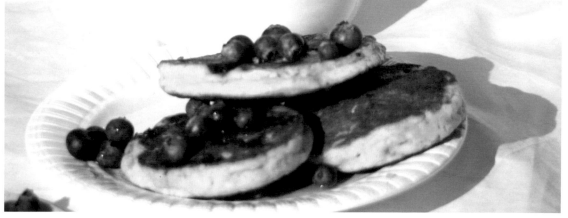

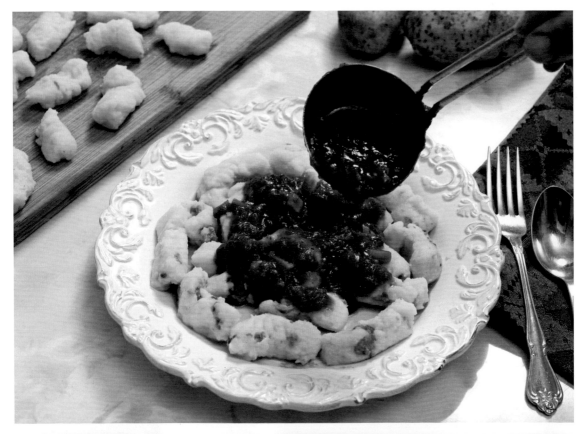

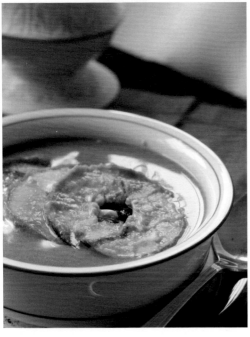

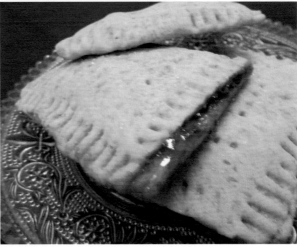

TOP Marinara Sauce with Potato and Italian Sausage Gnocchi, page 135

BOTTOM LEFT Pumpkin Soup with Apple Croutons, page 89

BOTTOM RIGHT Morning Pastries (Toaster Tarts), page 18

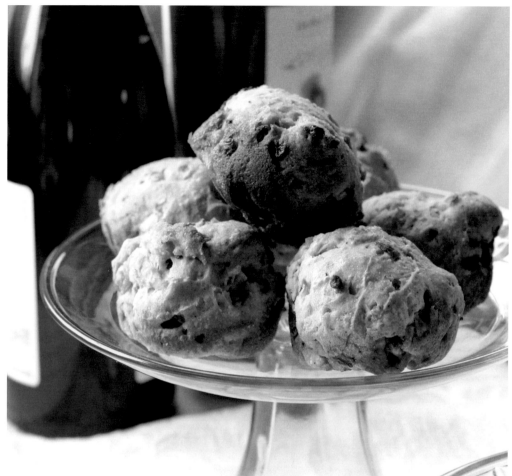

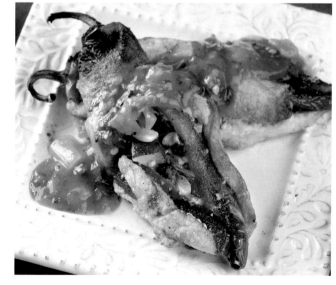

TOP Stuffing Rolls, page 69

BOTTOM Chili Rellenos, page 41

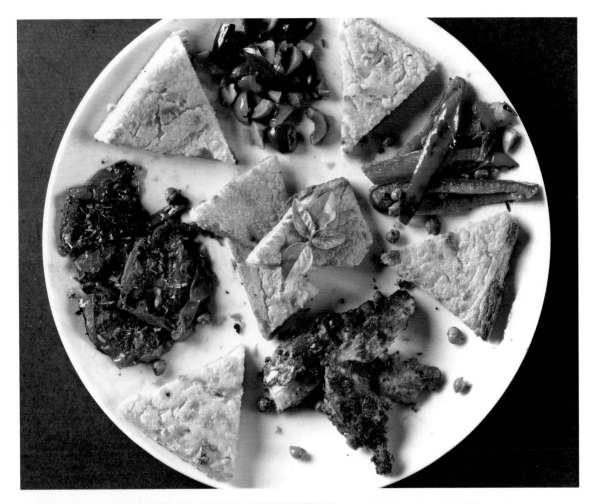

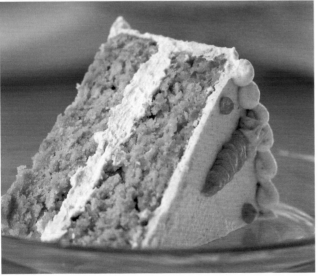

TOP Chickpea Crostini with Roasted Peppers, Tomato & Artichoke Toppings, page 40

BOTTOM Carrot Cake, page 161

BREAKFAST

&

BRUNCH

"Good nutrition is the key to a good life.
It gives us the energy to live life to its fullest."

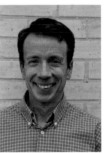

Recipes by
Matthew Kadey MSc, RD
and other celebrity chefs

Matthew Kadey

Waterloo, Ontario, Canada

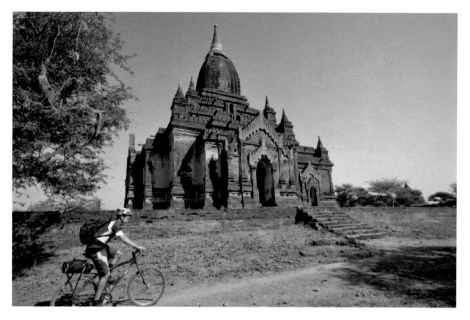

"Every cook needs inspiration. Mine comes via the bicycle."

Each year during the depths of the Canadian winter, I pack up and set off on a self-supported cycling slash eat-myself-silly-adventure through some far-flung (and warm) location. Every cook needs his or her inspiration, something that encourages them to experiment with new edibles, different food combinations and unfamiliar cooking techniques. Mine comes via the bicycle.

My food appetite often points me to my destination. When I was in the mood for fiery papaya salad, I booked a trip to Thailand. As a staunch supporter of all things coconut. I headed to the nation of Sri Lanka one year. (Who knew there were so many ways to make delicious vegetable curry?) It was while pedaling in Ethiopia that I was first exposed to injera, that ambrosial flatbread made with gluten-free teff. Teff's nutritional profile makes it a great breakfast grain. It can gussy up mundane pancakes and muffins and turn them into memorable morning fare.

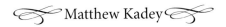

Upon returning from each excursion, I'm antsy to get back in the kitchen and rustle up new dishes that incorporate the international flavors from my trip.

As a registered dietitian, my role is to meet the menu requirements of those with special dietary needs. One way I accomplish this is to work with all-star gluten-free items like quinoa, millet, teff and brown rice flour. Developing gluten-free recipes is a great way to experiment with my cooking and broaden my culinary range and I try to encourage the same in others. I thoroughly enjoy amaranth porridge for breakfast and quinoa taboulleh for lunch.

Since science shows that eating foods in their less-processed forms can help us ward off a laundry list of chronic maladies, not to mention win the battle of the bulge, I naturally aspire to infuse my recipes with a panoply of whole foods. In their whole-food state, gluten-free items are nutritional bell ringers that contribute to our long-term well-being, making them even more enjoyable. Breakfast dishes can easily contain these nutrient-dense ingredients. In this form, the morning meal awakens our taste buds and presents itself as delightfully gourmet.

Matthew Kadey, MSc, RD, is a registered dietitian, nutrition writer and blogger and recipe developer. His nutrition and food features have appeared in dozens of publications, including *Living Without, Vegetarian Times, Men's Health, Runner's World, Shape, Prevention, Women's Health, Natural Health* and *Fit Pregnancy*. He received the James Beard Award for Food Journalism in 2013.

Kadey is the author of *Muffin Tin Chef* (Ulysses Press) and *The No-Cook No-Bake Cookbook* (Ulysses Press). Both contain recipes that can easily be adjusted to be gluten-free.

Where to find Matthew Kadey:

mattkadey.com
muffintinmania.com

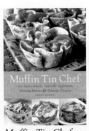
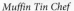

Muffin Tin Chef

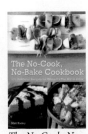

The No Cook, No Bake Cookbook

BREAKFAST AND BRUNCH

Matthew's
Maple Coconut Granola
Serves 6

Mixed with yogurt and berries, this tasty mixture of grains, seeds, spices and maple syrup makes for a knockout breakfast. Not just for the birds, nutritious gluten-free millet adds a twist to the time-honored oat-only granola. As with all granola recipes, this one is easy to customize based on your favorite seeds, dried fruit, spices and nuts, if tolerated.

Ingredients
2 cups gluten-free large-flake rolled oats
½ cup whole grain millet
½ cup flaked coconut
½ cup shelled pumpkin seeds (pepitas)
⅓ cup hemp seeds
½ cup dried cranberries or cherries
½ cup dried apricots, chopped
¼ cup cacao nibs, optional
1 teaspoon ground cinnamon
½ teaspoon allspice
¼ teaspoon salt
⅓ cup pure maple syrup, preferably dark grade
1 teaspoon fresh ginger, grated or very finely chopped
1 teaspoon pure vanilla extract

When making granola, be sure to choose large flake gluten-free rolled oats as opposed to the smaller quick-cook ones. See Shopping List on page 189 for brand suggestions.

Getting Started
Preheat oven to 275°F. Line a baking sheet with silicone or parchment paper.

Mixing the Ingredients
In a large bowl, combine oats, millet, coconut, pumpkin seeds, hemp seeds, cranberries, apricots, cacao nibs, cinnamon, allspice and salt. In a separate small bowl, combine maple syrup, ginger and vanilla. Add maple syrup mixture to oat mixture and mix until everything is moist. Stir in additional maple syrup if the mixture looks too dry.

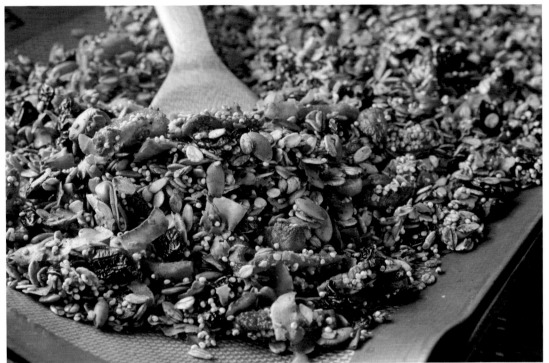
Maple Coconut Granola

To the Oven and Out

Spread out oat mixture on prepared baking sheet and cook for
1 hour or until golden brown, stirring every 15 to 20 minutes to
prevent burning. Cool completely and store in an airtight container
for up to 5 days.

Each serving contains 392 calories, 16g total fat, 6g saturated fat, 0g trans fat, 0mg cholesterol,
136mg sodium, 55g carbohydrate, 7g fiber, 24g sugars, 11g protein.

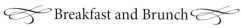
Matthew's
Quinoa Porridge with Cherry Sauce
Serves 4

Quinoa flakes are made by passing the grains through a roller to flatten them, making the flakes a perfect quick-cook breakfast alternative to oatmeal.

Ingredients
2 cups cherries, pitted and chopped
1 tablespoon honey
1½ teaspoons ground cinnamon, divided
1 teaspoon lemon zest
¾ cup water
1 teaspoon pure vanilla extract
1 teaspoon arrowroot powder or cornstarch, dissolved
in 2 tablespoons water
1½ cups hemp milk or milk of choice
2½ cups water
1½ cups quinoa flakes
1 large ripe banana, mashed
2 tablespoons ground flaxseed
⅓ cup raisins
⅓ cup raw sunflower seeds

Making the Cherry Sauce
In a small saucepan, bring cherries, honey, ½ teaspoon cinnamon, lemon zest and ¾ cup water to a boil. Reduce heat and simmer over low heat, stirring occasionally until cherries start to break down, about 5 minutes. Stir in vanilla and dissolved arrowroot; simmer 2 minutes more or until slightly thickened.

Making the Porridge
To make the porridge, place milk, 2½ cups water and remaining cinnamon in a medium saucepan. Bring to a boil. Add quinoa flakes and reduce heat, simmering 4 to 5 minutes or until most of the liquid has been absorbed and mixture is similar in consistency to cream of wheat. Stir occasionally. Stir in banana, flaxseed, raisins and sunflower seeds; heat 1 minute more. Place quinoa porridge in serving bowls and top with cherry sauce.

Each serving contains contains 413 calories, 13g total fat, 1g saturated fat, 0g trans fat, 0mg cholesterol, 54mg sodium, 67g carbohydrate, 9g fiber, 29g sugars, 11g protein.

Quinoa flakes are available at many health food stores and online.

When fresh cherries are out of season, look for frozen pitted cherries in the freezer section of your grocery store.

Reheat leftover porridge in a saucepan with a small amount of additional water or milk of choice.

Serve extra cherry sauce over yogurt or dairy-free ice cream.

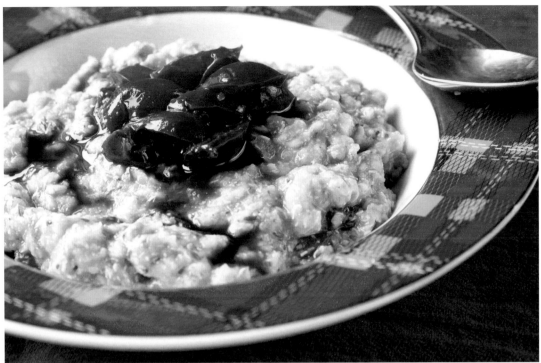

Quinoa Porridge with Cherry Sauce

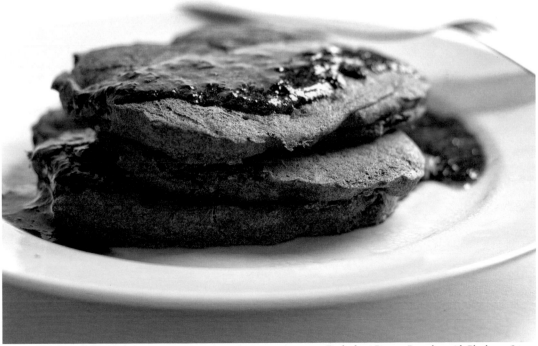

Buckwheat Banana Pancakes with Blueberry Sauce

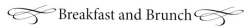

Matthew's
Buckwheat Banana Pancakes with Blueberry Sauce
Serves 2 to 3

Buckwheat flour infuses these hearty pancakes with extra protein, fiber and nutrients. If you find buckwheat's earthy flavor too strong on its own, replace half of it with another gluten-free flour, such as brown rice or quinoa. This recipe can be made egg-free.*

Ingredients
1 cup blueberries
¼ cup dark maple syrup or agave syrup
1 cup buckwheat flour
1 ripe banana, mashed
2 teaspoons baking powder
1 teaspoon ground cinnamon
¼ teaspoon salt
1 large egg*
⅔ cup + 1 tablespoon unflavored hemp milk or milk of choice

Making the Blueberry Sauce
To make blueberry sauce, whirl blueberries and maple syrup together in a blender until combined but still slightly chunky.

Mixing the Ingredients
In a large bowl, combine flour, banana, baking powder, cinnamon, salt and egg. Stir in milk. Add more milk if needed to reach desired consistency.

To the Stove
Lighty grease a non-stick skillet and heat over medium heat. Drop batter, ⅓ cup at a time, onto the skillet and cook 2 to 3 minutes per side, or until nicely browned. Serve pancakes topped with blueberry sauce.

*For **Egg-Free Pancakes,** omit 1 egg. Combine 1 tablespoon flax meal with 3 tablespoons hot water. Let sit 5 minutes until slightly thickened. Then add to recipe in place of 1 egg.

Each serving (3 pancakes) contains 324 calories, 4g total fat, 1g saturated fat, 0g trans fat, 70mg cholesterol, 562mg sodium, 70g carbohydrate, 7g fiber, 8g protein.

Matthew's
Coconut Black Rice Cereal
Serves 4

Creamy avocado adds a dose of heart-healthy monounsaturated fat. For best results, use coconut milk sold in tetra packs or cartons rather than the canned variety. Extra cooked black rice cereal can be stored in the refrigerator for up to 5 days.

Ingredients
2 cups water
1 cup uncooked black rice
1 teaspoon ground cinnamon
1 teaspoon ground ginger
2 tablespoons honey
1 teaspoon pure vanilla extract
2 cups coconut milk
1½ cups cubed pineapple or diced mango
1 ripe avocado, thinly sliced

Cooking the Rice
Place water, black rice, cinnamon and ginger into a medium-size saucepan. Bring to a boil. Reduce heat and simmer covered until all the water has been absorbed, about 30 minutes.

Stir in honey and vanilla. Let cool for 5 minutes. Taste and adjust sweetness, if desired.

To Serve
Divide cereal among 4 serving bowls and top with coconut milk, pineapple and avocado.

Fresh and dried fruit add natural sweetness to cereals. Many possess disease-thwarting antioxidants.

When using sweeteners, opt for less processed choices, such as honey, brown rice syrup, low-glycemic coconut palm sugar or pure maple syrup.

Warming spices, such as cinnamon, cloves, ginger and nutmeg, are the secret flavor boosters in cereal recipes. Bonus: They're virtually calorie-free and studies suggest diets heavy in spices are protective against several chronic diseases.

Each serving contains 552 calories, 33g total fat, 23g saturated fat, 0g trans fat, 0mg cholesterol, 20mg sodium, 35g carbohydrate, 5g fiber, 4g protein.

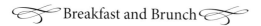

Matthew's
Orange Millet Cereal
Serves 4

When cooking grains like millet, try simmering them in different liquids, such as apple cider or orange juice, for a variety of flavor twists. A topping of naturally sweet coconut adds extra nuance.

Ingredients
1 cup millet
1¼ cups water
1 cup orange juice
¼ teaspoon ground cardamom
2 tablespoons honey
½ cup raisins or dried cranberries
⅓ cup raw sunflower seeds
2 cups hemp milk or milk of choice
¼ cup unsweetened shredded coconut

Cooking the Millet

Heat a medium-size saucepan over medium heat. Add millet and cook, stirring often, until it begins to brown and smells toasty, about 3 minutes.

Add water, orange juice and cardamom. Bring to a boil. Reduce heat and simmer covered for 30 minutes or until liquid has been absorbed and millet is tender.

Stir in honey, raisins and sunflower seeds. Let stand 5 minutes and then fluff with a fork.

To Serve

Divide cereal among 4 serving bowls. Top with milk and coconut.

When deciding what milk to pour over your cereal, consider hemp milk. It's allergy-friendly and provides more protein and omega fatty acids than most other plant milks.

Each serving contains 401 calories, 9g total fat, 2g saturated fat, 0g trans fat, 0mg cholesterol, 62mg sodium, 74g carbohydrate, 6g fiber, 9g protein.

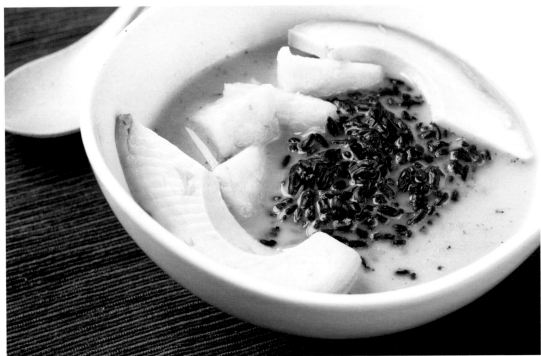

Coconut Black Rice Cereal with Pineapple and Avocado

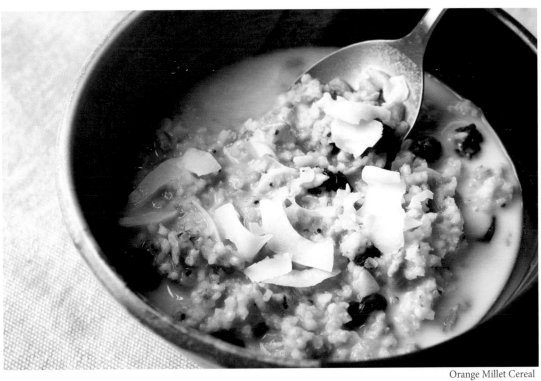

Orange Millet Cereal

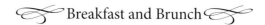

Teff Porridge
Serves 4
(RECIPE BY MATTHEW KADEY)

This rustic cereal is packed with heart-healthy fats and fiber from flax and pumpkin seeds to prevent mid-morning cravings. Reheat leftovers in a small saucepan with some additional water.

Ingredients
3½ cups + ⅓ cup water, divided
1 cup teff grain, preferably dark colored
1 teaspoon ground cinnamon
¼ teaspoon ground cloves
⅓ cup pumpkin seeds (pepitas) or hazelnuts, if tolerated
⅓ cup ground flaxseed, chia seeds or salba seeds
½ cup chopped dried pitted dates
1 teaspoon orange zest
1 banana, thinly sliced
¼ cup pure maple syrup, preferably dark grade

Cooking the Teff
In a medium-size saucepan, bring 3½ cups water to boil. Add teff, cinnamon and cloves and simmer for 12 minutes, stirring often to prevent clumping. Meanwhile, toast pumpkin seeds in a dry skillet over medium heat until they begin to pop and turn golden, about 3 minutes.

Stir flaxseed, dates, orange zest and additional ⅓ cup water into the teff. Heat for 5 minutes or until teff is tender.

To Serve
Divide teff among 4 serving bowls and top with toasted pumpkin seeds, banana and maple syrup.

Each serving contains 333 calories, 7g total fat, 1g saturated fat, 0g trans fat, 0mg cholesterol, 12mg sodium, 63g total carbohydrate, 11g fiber, 7g protein.

Incorporating unsaturated fats into your cereal bolsters flavor and makes it more of a complete meal. Found in seeds, flax, chia, avocado and nuts, these healthy fats help fend off coronary woes when consumed in moderate portions. They are also loaded with vital vitamins and minerals.

Airy Pancakes with Blueberries
Makes 16 3-inch pancakes
(RECIPE BY BETH HILLSON)

Serve these pancakes hot with real maple syrup or blueberry compote—or enjoy them plain. This recipe can be made with egg-free.*

Ingredients
2 cups *Living Without's* All Purpose Flour Blend (page xiv)
3 teaspoons baking powder
1½ teaspoons xanthan gum
½ teaspoon salt
⅓ cup sugar
3 large eggs,* separated
1½ cups milk or unflavored milk of choice
¾ teaspoon pure vanilla extract
6 tablespoons unsalted butter or non-dairy alternative, melted
1 cup fresh blueberries

Mixing the Ingredients
Combine flour blend, baking powder and sugar in a small bowl and set aside.

Separate the eggs. Place the yolks in a large mixing bowl. Add milk, vanilla and butter, whisking to combine.

Add the dry ingredients to the yolk mixture and whisk to blend.

In a separate bowl, beat egg whites until soft

peaks form. Do not overbeat; stop when you notice lines beginning to form and stay on the surface.

Fold half the beaten whites into the batter to blend. Fold remaining whites into the mixture. Do not blend completely. You should see bits of white foam in the batter.

On the Griddle and Off
Lightly oil a non-stick skillet and heat over medium heat.Using a ¼-cup scoop, drop batter onto preheated griddle. After batter has begun to set, sprinkle blueberries over the surface of each pancake. When the underside is golden brown, flip pancakes and cook until browned on the other side. Keep warm until served.

Each serving (3 pancakes) contains 472 calories, 19g total fat, 11g saturated fat, 0g trans fat, 169mg cholesterol, 778mg sodium, 66g carbohydrate, 4g fiber, 11g protein.

> *For **Egg-Free Airy Pancakes with Blueberries,** omit 3 eggs. Combine 3 tablespoons flax meal with 9 tablespoons hot water. Let sit for 5 minutes until slightly thickened. Add to wet ingredients to replace 3 ggs.

Homemade Breakfast Sausage
Makes 12 to15 patties
(RECIPE BY SUESON VESS)

Making your own sausage creates the flexibility to use fresh meat and seasonings of your choice. Plus, you avoid the artificial ingredients, preservatives and additives often seen in commercial brands. Adding dried or fresh fruit lends a hint of natural sweetness. This recipe is ideal for those who are following a rotation diet; make several batches, each with a different meat, and freeze it raw or precooked until ready to use.

Ingredients
1 pound ground dark turkey (or chicken, pork, beef or a combination)
1½ teaspoons marjoram or ½ teaspoon rubbed sage
½ teaspoon ground thyme
½ teaspoon salt
½ teaspoon ground white pepper
¼ teaspoon ground allspice
¼ teaspoon ground cinnamon
¼ teaspoon ground nutmeg
¼ teaspoon ground fennel seeds
⅛ teaspoon cayenne pepper, to taste
1 small pear or apple, cored and finely diced, optional (may leave skin on)
2 tablespoons dried cranberries or cherries, chopped, optional
Olive oil, grape seed oil or coconut oil, for sautéing

Mixing the Ingredients
In a large bowl, combine all ingredients until well blended.

Preparing and Cooking the Patties
Form mixture into 12 to 15 small patties with well-oiled hands.

Sauté patties in a large skillet over medium/medium-low heat with a small amount of oil for 2 to 3 minutes per side or until cooked through.

Serve hot. May be cooked and frozen for later use.

Each serving contains 65 calories, 3g total fat, 1g saturated fat, 0g trans fat, 24mg cholesterol, 3g carbohydrate, 106mg sodium, 1g fiber, 5g protein.

> To save steps, use 1 tablespoon Penzeys Breakfast/Pork Sausage Seasoning or Bavarian Seasoning (penzeys.com) in place of the 9 individual spices.

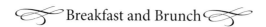

Breakfast Muffins with Fig Filling
Makes 15 muffins
(RECIPE BY REBECCA REILLY)

Loaded with fruit and fiber, these hearty favorites are ideal morning fare. This recipe can be made egg-free.*

Ingredients
2¾ cups *Living Without's* High-Protein
Flour Blend (page xiv)
¼ cup tapioca starch/flour
1 cup maple sugar or light brown sugar
1 tablespoon baking powder
1 tablespoon cream of rice cereal
½ teaspoon xanthan gum
⅛ teaspoon salt
1¼ cups warm milk of choice
⅓ cup oil of choice or unsweetened applesauce
2 large eggs*
1 teaspoon pure vanilla extract
Cinnamon sugar, optional

Filling
⅓ cup light brown sugar
½ teaspoon ground cinnamon
2 tablespoons butter or non-dairy alternative
⅓ cup orange juice
⅓ cup ground quick-cooking gluten-free oats
or quinoa flakes
1 cup dried figs, stems removed, fruit
cut into pieces

Getting Started
Preheat oven to 350°F. Lightly oil muffin tins or use muffin liners and lightly spray with cooking oil.

Mixing the Ingredients
Mix together flour blend, tapioca starch/flour, maple sugar, baking powder, cream of rice cereal, xanthan gum and salt in a large bowl.

In separate bowl, whisk together warm milk, oil, eggs and vanilla. Slowly incorporate wet mixture into dry ingredients and whisk until just smooth. Allow batter to sit for 5 minutes.

Making the Filling
To make filling, put all filling ingredients into a food processor and process until blended.

To the Oven and Out
Fill muffin tins half full with batter. Place a flattened teaspoon of filling on the batter and then scoop more batter on top to fill tins ¾ full.

Sprinkle batter with cinnamon sugar or Crumb Topping. Place in preheated oven and bake 18 to 20 minutes or until a sharp paring knife inserted in center comes out clean and hot to touch. Cool 10 minutes and remove from pan.

Each muffin contains 242 calories, 7g total fat, 1g saturated fat, 0g trans fat, 30mg cholesterol, 112mg sodium, 43g carbohydrate, 1g fiber, 14g sugars, 3g protein.

*For **Egg-Free Breakfast Muffins**, omit 2 eggs. Increase baking powder to 1½ tablespoons. Increase milk to 1½ cups. Increase oil or applesauce to ½ cup.

There'll be fig filling to spare. Use extra as a spread on gluten-free toast or biscuits.

Crumb Topping
Makes about 3 cups

Make your Breakfast Muffins extra-special by adding this Crumb Topping.

½ cup cold butter or non-dairy alternative
1 cup *Living Without's* All-Purpose Flour Blend
(page xiv)
1 cup brown sugar

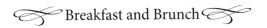

1 cup gluten-free oats
2 teaspoons ground cinnamon

Cut butter into small bits. Then combine all ingredients in a food processor and pulse until mixture forms into fine crumbs. Sprinkle over muffin batter and bake according to recipe directions.

Blueberry Breakfast Cookies
Makes 14 to 16
(RECIPE BY BETH HILLSON)

These cookies freeze well and can be reheated. If fresh blueberries are not available, use frozen, unthawed blueberries. This recipe can be made egg-free.*

Ingredients
2 cups *Living Without* High-Protein Flour Blend (page xiv)
⅓ cup packed light brown sugar, more for sprinkling on tops
1 tablespoon baking powder
½ teaspoon baking soda
1 teaspoon ground cinnamon
1 teaspoon xanthan gum
½ teaspoon salt
5 tablespoons cold unsalted butter or non-dairy alternative, cut into small pieces
2 large eggs*
½ cup yogurt or non-dairy yogurt, more for brushing tops
2 teaspoons pure vanilla extract
¾ cup fresh blueberries
¾ cup gluten-free crispy rice cereal

Getting Started
Preheat oven to 350°F. Line 2 cookie sheets with parchment paper.

Mixing the Ingredients
Thoroughly combine flour blend, brown sugar, baking powder, baking soda, cinnamon, xanthan gum, and salt in a large bowl. Cut in butter until mixture resembles coarse meal.

In a separate bowl, beat eggs, yogurt and vanilla for 1 minute. Add to dry ingredients and beat until smooth. Fold in blueberries and cereal.

Forming the Cookies
Scoop dough onto prepared cookie sheets, leaving about 1 inch between each cookie. Use plastic wrap to gently press and smooth cookies into ½ inch-thick disks. Brush with yogurt and sprinkle with brown sugar.

To the Oven and Out
Place in preheated oven and bake 19 to 20 minutes until done. Serve warm.

Each cookie contains 130 calories, 5g total fat, 3g saturated fat, 0g trans fat, 36mg cholesterol, 221mg sodium, 20g carbohydrate, 1g fiber, 3g protein.

*For **Egg-Free Breakfast Cookies,** omit 2 eggs. Add 1 tablespoon arrowroot to dry ingredients. Combine 1 tablespoon flax meal with 3 tablespoons hot water and let sit 5 minutes until thickened; use in place of eggs in recipe instructions.

These cookies come together quickly (25 minutes from start to finish) and they travel well. They freeze well, too.

Breakfast Egg Strata
Serves 4 to 6
(RECIPE BY SUESON VESS)

This easy, make-ahead breakfast casserole is great for busy mornings, entertaining or any time you want to wake up and have breakfast ready to pop into the oven. Start with the basic filling and vary the flavor by adding ingredients of your choice. For best results, do not replace the eggs in this recipe.

Ingredients
3-4 cups (4-5 slices) day-old gluten-free, dairy-free bread, cut into 1-inch cubes
6 large eggs
2 cups milk of choice
1 teaspoon ground mustard
1 teaspoon salt, to taste
1 teaspoon pepper, to taste
½ teaspoon dill weed, optional (adds buttery flavor without dairy or cheese)

Getting Started
Oil a 1-quart baking dish. Line dish with bread cubes. If desired, top bread with ingredients from 1 of the strata variations that follow this recipe.

Mixing the Ingredients
In a large bowl, whisk eggs with milk, ground mustard, salt, pepper and dill weed, if used.

Setting and Baking
Pour egg mixture over bread cubes and refrigerate 6 to 8 hours or overnight.

Preheat oven to 350°F. Place strata in preheated oven and bake 30 to 45 minutes until done.

Each serving contains 218 calories, 8g total fat, 2g saturated fat, 0g trans fat, 220mg cholesterol, 27g carbohydrate, 553mg sodium, 1g fiber, 9g protein.

For **Strata ala Benedict**, add:
½ cup gluten-free, dairy-free turkey bacon, cut into 1-inch pieces, or MSG-free, nitrate-free ham, cut into ¼-inch pieces
½ cup asparagus spears, par cooked and cut into 1-inch pieces

For **Strata Santa Fe**, add:
1 small can chopped green chilies
1 tomato, seeded, chopped
1 tablespoon fresh cilantro, chopped

Croissants
Makes 24 croissants
(RECIPE BY BETH HILLSON)

You'll love these light, luscious gluten-free pastries. Enjoy them plain, as the French do, or fill them with your favorite fruit spread. For best results, do not replace the eggs in this recipe.

Ingredients
1 cup sorghum flour
½ cup chickpea flour
½ cup almond meal or gluten-free flour of choice
1 cup white rice flour
1 cup cornstarch or tapioca starch/flour
4 teaspoons xanthan gum
1½ teaspoons salt
4 teaspoons active dry yeast
¼ cup sugar
1 cup warm milk of choice or water
2 large eggs
4 tablespoons (½ stick) butter or non-dairy alternative, melted
12 tablespoons (1½ sticks) cold butter or non-dairy alternative,* cut into small pieces
1 cup raspberry or other fruit preserves, optional
Egg wash (1 egg combined with 2 tablespoons cold water), optional

Mixing the Ingredients
In a large bowl, combine flours, xanthan gum and salt and blend well.

Scoop 1 cup of this flour mixture into a medium mixing bowl. Add yeast and sugar to this cup of flour mixture and blend thoroughly. Combine milk and eggs and add them to this mixture. Add melted butter and beat until smooth. Set aside.

Cut cold butter into remaining flour mixture until butter pieces are the size of large peas. Pour liquid batter into the flour and butter mixture and stir or beat until moistened throughout. Cover and refrigerate for 4 hours or overnight.

Working the Dough
Remove dough from refrigerator and press into a compact ball on a surface that has been lightly covered with rice flour. Divide dough into 3 equal parts. Roll** each third into a 12-inch circle with a rolling pin. Cut each circle into 8 pie-shaped wedges.

Separate wedges. Brush each wedge with gently warmed fruit preserves, if desired. Then roll up each wedge toward the point. Shape into a crescent by curving the edges.

Set croissants on an ungreased baking sheet or a sheet lined with parchment paper. Cover with plastic wrap and let them rise at room temperature until doubled. (This may take 2 hours if the room is cool.)

To the Oven and Out
Preheat oven to 400°F. Lightly brush each croissant wedge with egg wash, if desired. Place croissants in preheated oven and immediately lower oven temperature to 350°F. Bake 15 to 20 minutes or until golden.

Each croissant contains 178 calories, 10g total fat, 5g saturated fat, 0g trans fat, 39mg cholesterol, 20g carbohydrate, 159mg sodium, 1g fiber, 3g protein.

*If using non-dairy butter alternative, freeze it for 15 minutes before cutting it into small pieces.

**The thinner you roll out the wedges of dough, the more "layers" your croissants will have and the flakier they will be. However, dough should not be paper-thin.

Hot Cross Buns
Makes 9 buns
(RECIPE BY REBECCA REILLY)

This recipe is a delicious gluten-free version of the classic yeast rolls enjoyed during the Easter season. Icing drizzled across the top in an X is traditional, representing the cross. This recipe can be made egg-free.*

Ingredients
3 cups *Living Without's* High-Protein Flour Blend (page xiv), more as needed
⅓ cup sugar
4½ teaspoons (2 packages) rapid-rise yeast
½ cup dry milk powder or non-dairy milk powder
3 teaspoons xanthan gum
1 teaspoon salt
1 tablespoon ground cinnamon
1 cup warm water (110°F–115°F)
¼ cup light olive oil or melted coconut oil
3 large eggs, lightly beaten*
1 teaspoon cider vinegar
1 cup raisins
¼ cup diced candied lemon peel, optional
¼ cup diced candied orange peel, optional
3 tablespoons melted butter or shortening of choice, for brushing

Getting Started
Lightly grease a 10-inch round cake pan.

Mixing the Ingredients
Mix flour blend, sugar, yeast, powdered milk,

xanthan gum, salt and cinnamon together. Add water, oil, eggs and vinegar and beat for 5 minutes. Mix in raisins and candied fruit peels, if desired. If needed, add additional flour blend, (one spoonful at a time) until dough is easy to handle.

Working the Dough
Scrape dough onto a floured cookie sheet. Cut dough into 8 or 9 pieces and gently shape each into a ball. Place 1 ball of dough in the center of prepared cake pan. Loosely arrange the remaining balls around it, leaving room for buns to rise. Brush the buns with melted butter and cut an X into the top of each bun. Cover with a piece of plastic wrap and let rise in a warm, draft-free spot for 20 to 30 minutes. Meanwhile, preheat the oven to 375°F.

To the Oven and Out
Place buns in preheated oven and bake for 25 to 30 minutes until golden brown. Remove from oven and cool on a rack. When the buns are cool, drizzle icing over the scored X.

Each bun contains 467 calories, 13g total fat, 8g saturated fat, 0g trans fat, 81mg cholesterol, 296mg sodium, 84g carbohydrate, 4g fiber, 7g protein.

Icing
Makes 1½ cups
1½ cups confectioners' sugar, sifted
2 tablespoons milk of choice
¼ teaspoon pure vanilla extract

Whisk confectioners' sugar, milk and vanilla together until smooth. Add more milk if icing is too thick.

*For **Egg-Free Hot Cross Buns**, omit 3 eggs. Combine 4½ tablespoons applesauce + 1½ teaspoons baking powder + 2¼ teaspoons

Ener-G egg replacer + 3 tablespoons water in a blender. Blend briefly until frothy. Mix with wet ingredients and proceed with the recipe.

Morning Pastries (Toaster Tarts)
Makes 12 pastries
(RECIPE BY REBECCA REILLY)

Kids love these fruit-filled tarts, a gluten-free version of the ever-popular Pop-Tarts® breakfast treats. This recipe can be made egg-free.*

Ingredients
2⅓ cups *LivingWithout's* High-Protein Flour Blend (page xiv)
2½ teaspoons baking powder
1½ teaspoons xanthan gum
¼ teaspoon salt
⅓ cup sugar
6 tablespoons vegetable shortening or butter
2 large eggs*
1 teaspoon cider vinegar
Fruit jam, preserves or fruit butter, for filling (heat briefly in microwave for easier spreading)
1 large egg yolk** mixed with 2 tablespoons milk of choice, or ¼ cup milk of choice, for brushing tops
Sugar, for sprinkling, optional

Getting Started
Preheat oven to 350°F. Grease a cookie sheet and set aside.

Mixing the Ingredients
Mix together flour blend, baking powder, xanthan gum and salt in a medium bowl.

In a separate bowl, cream together sugar and shortening, beating until light.

Beat in 2 eggs until creamy. Add vinegar and blend. Then stir in the dry ingredients to make a soft dough. Wrap dough in plastic wrap and refrigerate 10 to 15 minutes.

Working the Dough
Divide the dough in half. Cover half with plastic wrap and refrigerate. Roll the other half into a rectangle about ¹⁄₁₆-inch thick. (For easy rolling, cut a large zip-top plastic bag in half along the seams and roll dough out between the 2 pieces.) Even out the edges of the dough and cut it into 3x5-inch rectangles.

Spread 1 heaping teaspoon of warm jam evenly over each dough rectangle, leaving a generous margin. Brush margins with egg-yolk mixture, or milk of choice.

Fold dough rectangles in half, leaving jam inside. Press edges together and crimp with the tines of a fork. Place pastry on prepared cookie sheet, pricking top with a fork. For a shiny finish and golden color, brush tops with egg yolk mixture, if desired. Sprinkle with sugar, if desired. Repeat with remaining dough.

To the Oven and Out
Place pastries in preheated oven and bake for 15 minutes, just until edges are browned. During baking, prick them again one time to help keep them flat.

Remove from oven and cool. Wrap and store at room temperature or refrigerate.

Each serving contains 203 calories, 10g total fat, 6g saturated fat, 0g trans fat, 68mg cholesterol, 195mg sodium, 26g carbohydrate, 1g fiber, 3g protein.

*For **Egg-Free Morning Pastries,** omit 2 eggs. Combine 2 tablespoons flax meal with 6 tablespoons hot water. Let sit 5 minutes until thickened. Then add to recipe.

For frosted pastries, mix 1 cup confectioners' sugar with enough water or milk of choice to make an icing. Drizzle over top.

Spring Crepes with Blueberry Filling
Makes 8 crepes
(RECIPE BY SUESON VESS)

Folded in half, quartered or rolled, crepes are the perfect finger food. These thin, versatile pancakes work with sweet or savory fillings. Delicious with any fresh fruit, like Blueberry Filling, you can also stuff them with leftover veggies, such as sautéed spinach, cooked lentils or even mashed sweet potatoes with fresh chives. Try a crepe buffet and let guests make their own selection. For best results, do not replace the eggs in this recipe.

Ingredients
½ cup *Living Without's* All-Purpose
Flour Blend (page xiv)
½ cup milk of choice
¼ cup warm water
1½ tablespoons sugar
or 1 tablespoon honey or agave
¼ teaspoon salt
2 large eggs
2 tablespoons grape seed oil
or melted coconut oil, more for pan

Mixing the Ingredients
Combine all ingredients in a food processor and blend until smooth. Do not over-mix or batter will become foamy. Pour batter into a pitcher, cover and refrigerate for 30 minutes to 3 hours.

Making the Crepes
Using a paper towel, wipe the inside of a well-

seasoned 6- to 8-inch crepe pan, cast iron or non-stick skillet with a small amount of oil. Place pan over medium heat.

Stir the batter and pour 2 tablespoons into the pan, tilting to coat the bottom with a very thin layer of batter.

Cook just until the top is set and edges are slightly browned. Turn crepe over and cook the other side until it's lightly browned. Cook remaining crepes, stirring the batter before each one.

Serving or Saving

Place finished crepes between sheets of parchment or waxed paper to keep warm. Serve immediately or refrigerate for later use. Reheat gently in microwave or in preheated 325°F oven.

Each crepe contains 96 calories, 5g total fat, 1g saturated fat, 0g trans fat, 53mg cholesterol, 95mg sodium, 11g carbohydrate, 0g fiber, 3g sugars, 2g protein.

Blueberry Filling
Makes 4 cups

The blending of cooked and uncooked blueberries provides a wonderful mouth-feel that's both creamy and slightly chunky. For variation, try other berries or a combination of different berries mixed together.

Ingredients

4 cups fresh or frozen blueberries, divided
2 teaspoons cornstarch or arrowroot,
dissolved in ¼ cup cold water
1 tablespoon lemon juice
Sugar or natural sweetener, to taste,
optional

Making the Filling

Puree 1 cup berries in a blender or food proces-

sor, along with cornstarch/water mixture and lemon juice.

Pour puree into a saucepan and cook over medium heat for 2 to 3 minutes until thickened. Add 3 cups berries and sugar, to taste. Stir to combine.

Each ¼ cup serving contains 23 calories, 0g total fat, 0g saturated fat, 0g trans fat, 0mg cholesterol, 0mg sodium, 6g carbohydrate, 1g fiber, 0g protein

Pumpernickel Bagels
Makes 8 bagels
(RECIPE BY REBECCA REILLY)

Instant espresso and cocoa give these egg-free bagels a rich flavor.

Ingredients

Sweet rice flour, for dusting and rolling bagels
2 cups *Living Without's* High-Protein
Flour Blend (page xiv)
¾ cup sorghum flour
¼ cup gluten-free cornmeal
1 teaspoon salt
1½ teaspoons egg replacer
1 tablespoon xanthan gum
1 tablespoon rapid rise yeast
2 teaspoons toasted caraway seeds
2 tablespoons molasses
1 teaspoon cider vinegar
2 tablespoons vegetable oil
1 teaspoon gluten-free instant espresso
or powdered coffee
1 tablespoon unsweetened cocoa
1 cup warm water (110°F–115°F), more
as needed
1 teaspoon baking soda

Getting Started

Line a baking pan or cookie sheet with parch-

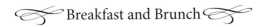
ment paper. Put some sweet rice flour on a second baking pan or cookie sheet.

Mixing the Ingredients
Put flour blend, cornmeal, salt, egg replacer, xanthan gum, yeast, sorghum flour, and caraway seeds into the bowl of a mixer and whisk together.

In a separate bowl, whisk together molasses, cider vinegar, oil, instant espresso, cocoa and 1 cup warm water.

Using the paddle attachment of the mixer, slowly incorporate liquid mixture into dry ingredients. Add more warm water, if necessary, to create a smooth consistency. Mixture should be quite thick. Beat on medium-high speed for 3 minutes.

Working the Dough and Boiling
To shape the bagels, drop a generous spoonful of batter onto the baking pan sprinkled with sweet rice flour. Lightly roll the dough in the flour to coat it and then shape it into a ball. Flatten ball slightly and then using your index finger, create a hole in the center, large enough so that it won't close up during rising and baking. Repeat with rest of the dough.

Place each bagel on parchment-lined cookie sheet. Lightly cover bagels with an oiled piece of plastic wrap and place them in a warm place to rise, about 15 to 20 minutes.

While bagels are rising, preheat oven to 375°F and bring a skillet of water to boil. Add baking soda to water.

Once bagels have risen, drop a few bagels into the boiling water. Simmer for 30 seconds, turn over and cook for another 30 seconds. Using a

slotted spoon, remove bagels, draining off water, and put bagels back on the same baking pan.

Top It Off
After bagels are boiled, brush them with an egg-wash (1 egg white beaten with 2 tablespoons cold water) or milk of choice. Then sprinkle each bagel lightly with sesame or caraway seeds, toasted onion, raw garlic bits, salt or topping of choice.

To the Oven and Out
Place bagels in preheated oven and bake 20 to 25 minutes until done. Cool on a rack.

Each bagel contains 257 calories, 5g total fat, 1g saturated fat, 0g trans fat, 0mg cholesterol, 305mg sodium, 50g carbohydrate, 3g fiber, 4g protein.

Sautéed Grits
Serves 8
(RECIPE BY JULES SHEPARD)

If you can't find gluten-free grits, pick up a package of gluten-free polenta. Polenta is made from ground yellow corn, rather than white. The color is a bit more yellow than grits but the taste and texture are similar. Leftover grits can be served with maple syrup for breakfast.

Ingredients
4 cups water
½ teaspoon sea salt
1 cup gluten-free quick-cooking grits
2 tablespoons butter or non-dairy alternative

Making the Grits
Bring water and salt to a boil in a large saucepan. Whisk in grits. Simmer, covered, for approximately 5 minutes or according to package directions.

Setting the Grits
When thickened, pour grits into a greased 9x9-inch baking pan. Smooth the top and refrigerate at least 2 hours until set. (It's best when refrigerated overnight.)

Flip the baking pan onto a large plate to remove the square of grits. Cut into 4 equal squares and then cut each square into two triangles.

Sautéing the Grits
In a cast iron pan or other skillet, melt the butter over medium heat. Add triangles of grits and gently sauté on each side until lightly browned and crispy.

Each serving contains 43 calories, 3g total fat, 2g saturated fat, 0g trans fat, 8mg cholesterol, 121mg sodium, 4g carbohydrate, 0g fiber, 0g protein.

> For **Cheese Grits,** stir in shredded cheese (dairy or non-dairy) while grits are simmering.
>
> For **Savory Grits,** add chopped peppers, cooked bacon bits and your favorite herbs while grits are simmering.
>
> For **Breakfast Casserole,** toss cooked grits with scrambled eggs or sautéed tofu, if tolerated, shredded cheese (dairy or non-dairy), salt and pepper. Bake in a greased casserole dish at 325°F for 20 minutes or until cheese is melted throughout.
>
> For **Mush,** pour grits into a high-sided pan and refrigerate overnight. Slice thinly and fry until crispy and golden. Serve with pure maple syrup.
>
> For **Fried Grits,** slice cold grits into thick strips, like steak fries. Roll in beaten egg or milk of choice and then in gluten-free flour. Shake off excess. Fry in ½-inch-deep hot oil, flipping to fry both sides until golden brown. Drain on paper towels. Serve hot.

Savory Zucchini Pancakes
Serves 4 to 6
(RECIPE BY SUESON VESS)

These quick, nutritious pancakes are an easy way to put "green" on your breakfast plate. Top with dairy-free sour cream or yogurt. This recipe can be made egg free.*

Ingredients
2 medium zucchini
½ teaspoon salt
2 large eggs*
2 tablespoons gluten-free flour of choice**
1 tablespoon fresh dill weed or 1 teaspoon dried dill weed
¼ teaspoon ground pepper
1 small onion, finely minced or grated
2 tablespoons coconut or olive oil, for sautéing

Mixing the Ingredients
Grate zucchini and toss with salt. Put salted zucchini onto a clean cotton dish towel and squeeze out extra liquid.

In a large bowl, whisk together eggs, flour, dill and pepper. Stir in zucchini and onion.

Cooking the Pancakes
Place a small amount of oil in a large skillet or non-stick griddle over medium heat. If using an electric griddle, heat pan to 300°F to 325°F.

Spoon 3 to 4 tablespoons (a ladle works nicely) of zucchini mixture onto the hot griddle.

Flatten pancakes slightly with spatula. Cook 2 to 3 minutes on each side or until golden and cooked through. Add additional oil as needed between batches.

Each serving contains 490 calories, 6g total fat, 1g saturated fat, 0g trans fat, 70mg cholesterol, 224mg sodium, 4g carbohydrate, 1g fiber, 3g protein.

*For **Egg-Free Savory Zucchini Pancakes,** omit 2 eggs. Combine 2 tablespoons flax meal with 6 tablespoons hot water. Let sit 5 minutes until slightly thickened. Then add to recipe in place of eggs.

**Use a gluten-free flour blend or a single flour, such as sorghum flour, sweet rice flour or tapioca starch/flour.

Vegetable Quiche
Serves 6 to 8
(RECIPE BY SUESON VESS)

Coconut milk makes this quiche creamy. You won't miss the cheese. Do not pre-bake the pie crust before filling. For best results, do not replace the eggs in this recipe.

Ingredients
1 cup canned coconut milk (not light)
4 large eggs
1 teaspoon ground mustard
¼ teaspoon salt
¼ teaspoon pepper
1 tablespoon olive oil or coconut oil
3 cups chopped vegetables (leeks, sweet bell peppers, zucchini, asparagus, mushrooms, broccoli, spinach, kale, etc.)
1 (8-inch or 9-inch) gluten-free, dairy-free pie crust, unbaked
1 tablespoon chives or green onion tops
¼-½ teaspoon tarragon

Getting Started
Preheat oven to 350°F.

Mixing the Ingredients
Whisk together coconut milk, eggs, ground

mustard, salt and pepper. Set aside.

Preparing the Vegetables
Add oil to a large skillet. Sauté vegetables over medium heat until just softened, about 3 to 5 minutes.

Put sautéed vegetables into unbaked pie crust. Add egg mixture and sprinkle with chives and tarragon.

Baking the Quiche
Bake quiche in preheated oven for 45 minutes or until done. A knife inserted in center of filling should come out clean.

Each serving contains 277 calories, 14g total fat, 10g saturated fat, 0g trans fat, 141mg cholesterol, 31g carbohydrate, 271mg sodium, 5g fiber, 9g protein.

APPETIZERS

"When it comes to appetizers, there's no right or wrong. Make a few for a small gathering or make a lot and throw a party. Just hold the gluten and dairy so all can enjoy."

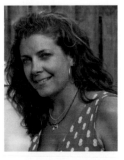

Recipes by
Jules Dowler Shepard
and other celebrity chefs

Jules Dowler Shepard

Baltimore, Maryland

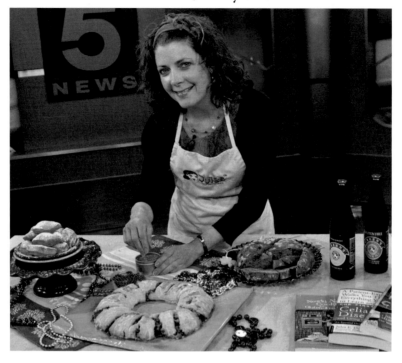

"Every recipe can be gluten-free as long as you start with a good flour blend."

Afterwards years of being plagued with unexplained illness, I was diagnosed with celiac disease in 1999. The food limitations seemed overwhelming but I was determined to prove to myself that gluten-free living could be delicious and varied, too. So I began experimenting in the kitchen.

As a lifelong baker, I knew I needed a good flour replacement that would mimic the Gold Medal flour I grew up with. It had to contain the right balance of starches and whole-grain flours in order to minimize grittiness and produce light-textured baked goods. I experimented until I developed the blend that behaved like gluten-filled flour and worked in all my favorite recipes. From that flour blend, the company Jules Gluten Free was born and the idea for my first cookbook took hold.

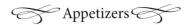

I found not only my health but my passion. I gave up my career as a prosecuting attorney and devoted my time to baking and teaching gluten-free cooking classes. And every time I baked, my family got to eat the results. That's not a bad way to live.

With more than a decade of experience in a gluten-free kitchen, I firmly believe that every recipe can be made gluten-free as long as you start with a good flour blend that has the right balance of starches and flours.

Don't be daunted by the switch to gluten-free living. It is not difficult. Just approach this lifestyle one recipe at a time. And remember, everyone makes mistakes in the kitchen—everyone. Most are not ruin-your-day mistakes, so don't toss something that didn't turn out as you'd hoped. Think about how it can be repurposed. A sunken loaf of bread can be bread pudding or bread crumbs. A fallen cake can be disguised with a nice, thick layer of frosting. Crumbly cookies can make wonderful ice cream toppings. It's all in what you make of it!

Jules Shepard lectures and gives gluten-free baking demonstrations all over the United States. She heads product and recipe development at Jules Gluten Free, a company specializing in gluten-free flour and baking mixes. In her spare time, Shepard advocates for those with celiac disease and gluten-related disorders, including lobbying for a national gluten-free labeling regulation. In May 2011 in Washington DC, she and other passionate volunteers constructed the world's tallest gluten-free cake to bring attention to the need for gluten-free labeling through the organization she co-founded, 1in133.org.

Shepard is author of *Nearly Normal Cooking for Gluten Free Eating* (BookSurge Publishing, LLC), *The First Year: Celiac Disease and Living Gluten Free* (Da Capo Press) and *Free For All Cooking* (Da Capo Press).

Where to find Jules Shepard:
julesglutenfree.com

These books are available at LivingWithout.com

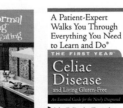
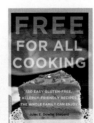

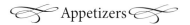

Appetizers

Jules's
Hoppin' John Hush Puppies
Serves 8

At the stroke of midnight on New Year's Eve, folks in the South can often be found enjoying a culinary tradition that ought not be kept a secret, "Hoppin' John." Stories of the origins of this rice and black-eyed pea dish are nearly as varied as the recipes bearing its name. People hailing from many regions have enjoyed hush puppies for centuries—as will your family and guests.

Ingredients
2 cups black-eyed peas, dried and soaked, canned or frozen
1 tablespoon extra virgin olive oil
¾ cup carrots, peeled and diced
½ cup celery, diced
1 small red onion, diced
1 teaspoon minced garlic
¼ cup dry white wine
1 cup cooked brown rice
2 tablespoons fresh Italian parsley, chopped
1 gluten-free smoked chipotle pepper in adobo sauce, diced
1 teaspoon sea salt
1 teaspoon cracked black pepper
1 tablespoon *Living Without's* All-Purpose Flour Blend (page xiv)
Oil, for frying

Getting Started
If using dried peas, drain after soaking. For dried or frozen peas, place in a large pot and cover with water. Bring to a boil. Then lower to simmer, uncovered, for 45 minutes or until tender. Add more water during the simmer if the water level reduces to below the peas.

Once cooked and tender, drain and set aside. If using canned peas, rinse, drain and set aside without cooking.

If using dried peas, rinse and soak them overnight and then rinse them again. Cover peas with 2 inches of water, bringing them to boil in a large pot. Cover pot and reduce heat to a simmer for about 3 hours, testing for doneness regularly.

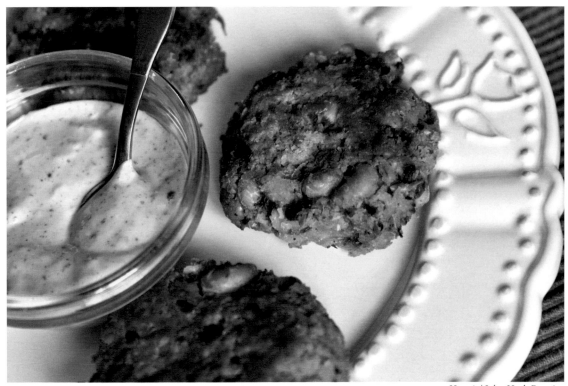

Hoppin' John Hush Puppies

Sautéeing the Vegetables
In a large skillet, heat olive oil over medium heat. Add carrots, celery and onion and sauté for 10 minutes or until the onion is translucent.

Add garlic and cook another 2 minutes. Add the wine and stir. Continue to cook over low heat until the wine has evaporated and mixture is fairly dry. Set aside.

Making the Pea Mash
Measure 2 cups of the prepared peas and set aside. Pour remaining peas into a large mixing bowl and blend with a paddle attachment or mash with a potato masher until the peas lose their definition and a sticky mash is formed.

Putting It Together
Fold in the sautéed vegetables, rice, Italian parsley, chipotle pepper, salt and pepper until fully integrated. Stir in the flour. Gently fold in the remaining peas, taking care to preserve some of them whole. Cover and chill for 30 minutes to 1 hour.

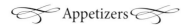

Forming and Frying the Patties

Once chilled, scoop 1 to 2 tablespoons of the mixture into your hands and form into hush puppy-shaped barrels or flattened patties, approximately ½-inch thick.

Heat oil in a deep fryer or deep pot for hush puppies. Fill pot with enough oil to cover the entire hush puppy. For frying patties, add oil to a heavy skillet, covering the skillet bottom with oil. Place puppies or patties gently into oil heated to medium-high, and turn or flip them when browned on 1 side, approximately 2 to 3 minutes per side. Drain them on paper towels.

To the Table

Serve with Lemon Dijon Aioli Sauce.

Lemon Dijon Aioli Sauce

Makes ½ cup

½ cup gluten-free, dairy-free mayonnaise

2 teaspoons lemon juice

2 teaspoons Dijon mustard

½ teaspoon minced garlic

¼ teaspoon cayenne pepper

Making the Sauce

Stir ingredients together in a small bowl. Refrigerate until cold and serve with warm or cold Hoppin' John Hush Puppies.

> If using canned black-eyed peas, rinse and drain before adding them to the recipe.

> For a list of companies offering gluten-free, dairy-free, egg-free mayonnaise, see Shopping List, page 189.

Each serving of hush puppies without sauce contains 172 calories, 7g total fat, 1g saturated fat, 0g trans fat, 4mg cholesterol, 444mg sodium, 22g carbohydrate, 4g fiber, 4g sugars, 5g protein.

Each serving of sauce contains 59 calories, 5g total fat, 1g saturated fat, 0g trans fat, 4mg cholesterol, 121mg sodium, 49g carbohydrate, 0g fiber, 1g sugars, 0g protein.

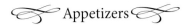

Jules's
Spaghetti Squash Latkes
Serves 6

One night, I found myself with no menu, only a spaghetti squash and a hankering for latkes. Although latkes have come to mean "potato pancakes," this dish can be made with nearly anything. So here's a version that uses spaghetti squash instead of potatoes.

Squash is naturally gluten-free and dairy-free. I cooked the winter squash and combed through it to gather my "noodles" for this great-tasting appetizer. It also makes a tasty side or a light vegetarian lunch. This recipe can be made egg-free.*

Ingredients

1 medium spaghetti squash (to yield 1 pound cooked, combed "noodles")
1 egg*
3 tablespoons *Living Without's* All-Purpose Flour Blend (page xiv)
2 teaspoons diced green chili peppers
1-2 gluten-free chipotle peppers in adobo sauce, diced
1 teaspoon sea salt
½ teaspoon cracked black pepper
1 tablespoon olive oil, for frying
Salsa, sour cream or non-dairy alternative, hummus, black beans or refried beans, as condiments

Getting Started
Preheat oven to 375°F.

Cut squash in half and remove strings and seeds. Lay each half, cut side down, on a baking pan with enough water to cover the surface of the pan.

Baking and Working the Squash
Bake in preheated oven for 30 minutes or until fork tender (cooking time will vary depending on the size of your squash). The skin will start to bubble a bit when it is done. Remove from the oven and allow to sit until it is cool enough to handle.

Combing the Squash
Comb through the cut sides of the cooked squash from top to bottom with a fork, creating lengths of "noodles."

Gluten-free brands of chipotle peppers in adobo sauce, like La Morena and La Costeña, are available in the ethnic foods aisle of large supermarkets. Read labels carefully.

Spaghetti squash makes a fat-free, low-carb, low-calorie "pasta" that is full of vitamins.

*For **Egg-Free Spaghetti Squash Latkes,** omit 1 egg Combine 1 tablespoon flax meal with 3 tablespoons warm water. Let sit for 5 minutes until slightly thickened. Add to other ingredients in place of the egg.

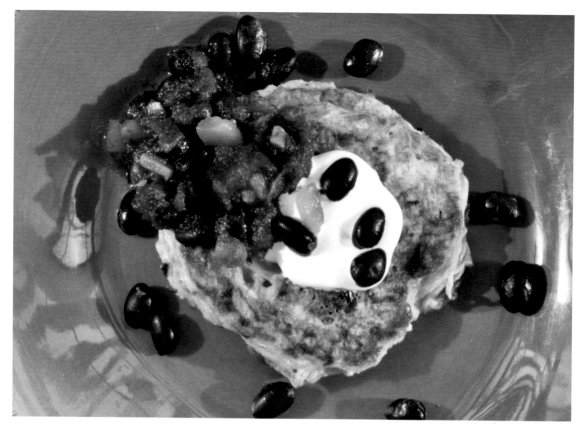

Spaghetti Squash Latke

Combining the Ingredients

Measure out 1 pound of "noodles" to a large bowl. Mix in beaten egg, flour, chili peppers, diced chipotle pepper, salt and pepper. The mixture should hold together well. Drain in a colander if it is watery.

Finishing Up

Heat 1 tablespoon of oil in a large skillet over medium-high heat. Spoon heaping tablespoons of the latke mixture onto the hot oil and gently flatten to an approximately 3-inch diameter. Fry until lightly browned. Then flip to fry on the other side.

To the Table

Remove cooked latkes to a foil-lined baking sheet and keep warm in a 200°F oven until ready to serve.

Each serving contains 48 calories, 1g total fat, 0g saturated fat, 0g trans fat, 35mg cholesterol, 434mg sodium, 8g carbohydrate, 1g fiber, 2g sugars, 2g protein.

To reheat these latkes, use an oven or toaster oven. They will lose their crispness if warmed in a microwave.

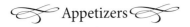

Jules's
Black Bean Chipotle Chili in Masa Cups
Serves: 10

These easy-to-serve, bite-size masa cups filled with hearty chili render silverware unnecessary. Spice chili up or down, according to your taste. The beautiful thing about chili is that there is no wrong way to make it. This recipe makes more than enough to fill 24 masa cups. Use extra as a dip for corn tortilla chips. Masa cups can be made egg-free.*

Chili Ingredients
3 tablespoons extra virgin olive oil
4 carrots, peeled and diced
1 large yellow onion, chopped
2 celery stalks, diced
1½ teaspoons minced garlic
1-2 gluten-free chipotle peppers in adobo sauce, diced
2 teaspoons chili powder
2 teaspoons cumin
1-2 teaspoons chipotle seasoning
Salt and cracked pepper, to taste
1 (28-ounce) can whole peeled tomatoes or
11-12 large tomatoes, peeled
2 (15-ounce) cans black beans, rinsed and drained
2 cups gluten-free beer
2 tablespoons minced fresh cilantro

Getting Started
Heat olive oil in a large pot over medium-high heat. Add the diced carrots, onions and celery, sautéing until onions are translucent. Add garlic, diced chipotle peppers and spices.

Puréeing the Tomatoes
Purée tomatoes in a large food processor or blender. (If using fresh tomatoes, peel them by dipping in boiling water for 30 seconds and then immersing in ice water until cooled. Peel off the loosened skin once the tomatoes have cooled.)

Putting It Together
Add purée to the sautéed vegetables. Then add the drained black beans. Pour in the beer and add cilantro, stirring well.

Use extra chili as a dip for gluten-free tortilla chips.

If using dried beans, prepare them according to package instructions before adding to this recipe.

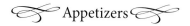

Finishing Up

Simmer chili uncovered until all vegetables are tender and chili has cooked down to desired consistency. It should not be watery when served in Masa Cups.

Masa Cups
Makes 24

½ cup cream cheese or non-dairy alternative, room temperature
½ cup butter or non-dairy alternative, room temperature
1 large egg*
1¼ cups *Living Without's* All Purpose Flour Blend (page xiv)
¾ cup masa harina
1 teaspoon baking powder
½ teaspoon sea salt
Cilantro leaves, for garnish

Getting Started

Preheat oven to 350°F. Lightly grease 24 mini-muffin cups.

Mixing It All Together

Beat together the cream cheese and butter in a large bowl. Once creamed, add the egg and beat until incorporated. Add dry ingredients and whip together until blended.

Making the Masa Cups

Spoon tablespoons of dough into the palms of your hands and form into 24 individual balls. Gently shape the balls into disks. Press individually into the bottom and up the sides of prepared muffin cups, taking care to cover the entire cup with dough and keeping the dough uniformly thin, no more than ¼-inch thick.

Finishing Up

Bake in preheated oven for 18 minutes. Set aside to cool before serving. Spoon chili (cooled or hot) into each muffin cup. Garnish with cilantro leaves and serve.

*For Egg-Free Masa Cups, combine 1 tablespoon flax meal with 3 tablespoons warm water. Let sit for 5 minutes until thickened. Add flax meal mixture to creamed cream cheese and butter and proceed with recipe.

Each masa cup with chili contains 124 calories, 6g total fat, 3g saturated fat, 0g trans fat, 21mg cholesterol, 222mg sodium, 15g carbohydrate, 2g fiber, 3g protein.

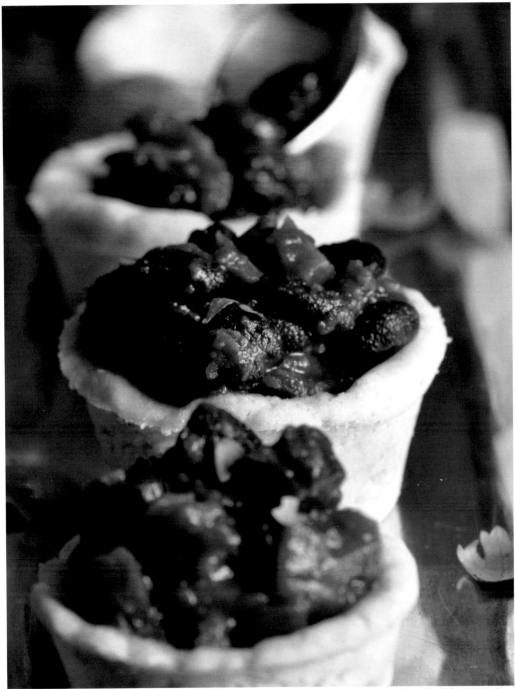

Black Bean Chipotle Chili in Masa Cups

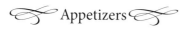

Jules's
Watermelon Salsa
Serves 10

Think fresh. Think cold. Think refreshing. Think flavor. That pretty much describes this yummy salsa, the perfect addition to any warm-weather occasion. Add spice if you wish or keep it mild. Keep chips at the ready to taste-test as you go (bonus!). Double or triple the recipe if you're serving a large group.

Ingredients
3 cups seeded or seedless watermelon, diced (about ¼ of a watermelon)
½ cup chopped fresh or grilled bell pepper
1 ear grilled or boiled corn
2 tablespoons fresh lime juice
1 tablespoon chopped cilantro leaves
1 tablespoon chopped green onion
2 tablespoons diced green chili peppers

For more heat, use diced jalapeño peppers instead of green chili peppers.

Making the Salsa
Chop and dice ingredients. Mix well in a large bowl. Cover and refrigerate until served.

Each serving contains 29 calories, 0g total fat, 0g saturated fat, 0g trans fat, 0mg cholesterol, 3mg sodium, 7g carbohydrate, 1g fiber, 4g sugars, 1g protein.

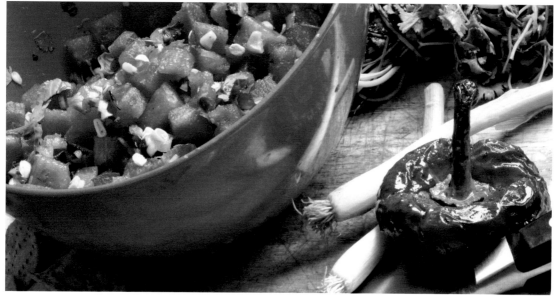

Watermelon Salsa

PHOTO BY JEFF RASMUSSEN

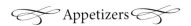

Jules's
Mini Quiche Poppers
Makes 48

Vary this versatile appetizer to suit your menu. There's no need to make time-consuming crusts. The gluten-free flour settles to the bottom for a crust that holds quiches together beautifully. For best results, do not replace the eggs in this recipe.

Ingredients
1-2 tablespoons extra virgin olive oil
1 cup mixed diced raw vegetables*
4 eggs, lightly beaten
1 cup sour cream or non-dairy alternative
1 cup cheddar cheese or non-dairy alternative
2 cups shredded mozzarella, Monterey Jack or non-dairy mild white cheese
¼ cup *Living Without's* All-Purpose Flour Blend (page xiv)
1 teaspoon chopped Italian parsley
1 teaspoon dried oregano
1 teaspoon dried basil
Pinch salt
1 teaspoon cracked black pepper
Grape tomatoes, sliced, for garnish

*Try sliced mushrooms, peas, corn, broccoli pieces, diced zucchini, bell peppers, asparagus, onion, red potatoes, wilted spinach or any other vegetables of your choosing.

Getting Started
Preheat oven to 350°F. Generously grease mini-muffin tins (enough for 48).

Sautéing the Vegetables
In a large pan, heat olive oil to medium-high. Sauté vegetables of your choice, cooking potatoes longer than any other addition. Set aside to cool.

Making the Filling
Combine eggs, sour cream, cheeses, flour, herbs, salt and pepper in a large mixing bowl and beat well. Stir in sautéed ingredients. Spoon mixture into prepared mini-muffin tins to two-thirds full. Top with 1 grape tomato slice on each mini quiche.

Finishing Up
Bake in preheated oven for approximately 25 minutes or until the centers

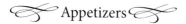
are no longer jiggly and a knife inserted into quiche comes out mostly clean. Cool for 10 minutes before removing and serving.

Each quiche popper contains 58 calories, 4g total fat, 2g saturated fat, 0g trans fat, 29mg cholesterol, 89mg sodium, 2g carbohydrate, 0g fiber, 4g protein.

Jules's
Pumpkin Pepper Hummus
Makes 2½ cups

Hummus has become a familiar condiment and is now available in all kinds of flavors. Making your own hummus is much easier than you might think, and there are benefits besides better taste and lower cost. Homemade allows you to tailor the recipe to your own liking—add more garlic or less, add red pepper or not—adjust the seasonings to suit your palate.

Ingredients
1 (15-ounce) can chickpeas, rinsed and drained
5 tablespoons pure pumpkin purée
¼ cup roasted red peppers
3 tablespoons lemon juice
2 tablespoons extra virgin olive oil
2 tablespoons sunflower seeds, hulled
½ teaspoon coarse sea salt
¼ teaspoon minced garlic
Allspice, to sprinkle on top

Making the Hummus
Combine all ingredients except allspice in the bowl of a large food processor. Purée until smooth.

Finishing Up
Spoon dip into a serving bowl and sprinkle with allspice.

If using canned pumpkin, make sure to pick unflavored pure pumpkin purée. Some canned pumpkin contains spices and other additives more suited to pumpkin pie recipes.

Each tablespoon contains 22 calories, 1g total fat, 0g saturated fat, 0g trans fat, 0mg cholesterol, 94mg sodium, 3g carbohydrate, 1g fiber, 1g protein.

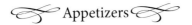

Apricot Chicken Wings
Serves 6 to 10
(RECIPE BY SUESON VESS)

These wings are crowd pleasers. Turmeric, a spice that naturally reduces inflammation, ups the health benefits without altering the flavor. Serve warm or at room temperature.

Ingredients
⅓ cup gluten-free soy sauce or wheat-free tamari
1 (8-ounce) jar apricot preserves, preferably fruit juice sweetened
3-4 tablespoons rice vinegar
½ teaspoon garlic powder
½ teaspoon turmeric
¼ teaspoon cayenne pepper, or to taste
2 tablespoons tapioca starch/flour
3 pounds chicken wings (cut into pieces at joints)

Making the Marinade
To make marinade, combine soy sauce, preserves, rice vinegar, garlic powder, turmeric and pepper in a medium saucepan over medium heat. Mix tapioca starch/flour with an equal amount of water to make a slurry. Add to saucepan ingredients and continue cooking for 3 minutes, stirring continuously. Remove from heat and allow to cool.

Marinating the Chicken
In a zip-top plastic bag or glass container with tight-fitting lid, marinate chicken wings in apricot sauce for at least 4 hours or overnight in the refrigerator. Turn bag or container occasionally to distribute marinade thoroughly.

To the Oven and Out
Preheat oven to 375°F. Lightly grease a baking pan or line it with parchment paper.

Remove wings from refrigerator and place them in a single layer on prepared pan. Place in preheated oven and bake 40 minutes, turning and basting occasionally with accumulated juices.

Arrange on a platter and serve.

Each serving contains 367calories, 22g total fat, 6g saturated fat, 0g trans fat, 104mg cholesterol, 649mg sodium, 17g carbohydrate, 0g fiber, 26g protein.

Bacon-Wrapped Bleu Cheese Dates
Makes 24
(RECIPE BY ROBERT LANDOLPHI)

This hors d'oeuvre calls out sweet, salty, smoky and savory notes. Make a double batch, as these dates will disappear quickly.

Ingredients
24 dried, pitted dates
4 ounces bleu cheese or non-dairy alternative
12 strips bacon, halved crosswise

Getting Started
Preheat oven to 375°F. Line 2 baking sheets with parchment paper.

Stuffing and Wrapping the Dates
Cut a lengthwise slit in each date and stuff with 1 teaspoon bleu cheese. Squeeze the date shut and wrap tightly with bacon, using a toothpick to secure each date.

Baking the Dates
Place dates on prepared baking sheets, seam side down, and cook in preheated oven until bacon is crispy, about 12 to 15 minutes. Halfway through, turn dates over to cook evenly.

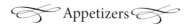

Finishing Up

Remove from oven. Allow dates to cool and serve at room temperature.

Each date contains 126 calories, 6g total fat, 2g saturated fat, 0g trans fat, 6mg cholesterol, 135mg sodium, 19g carbohydrate, 2g fiber, 2g protein.

Chickpea Crostini with Roasted Peppers, Tomato & Artichoke Toppings
Serves 8 to 10
(RECIPE BY MARY CAPONE)

This antipasto starts with a simple chickpea flatbread. Add roasted tomatoes, pan-fried artichoke hearts, roasted peppers and olives. Serve all ingredients on a large tray so that guests can help themselves. They'll have fun building their own crostini.

Chickpea Flatbread
1½ cups chickpea or garbanzo bean flour
2 cups warm water
4 tablespoons olive oil, divided, more for drizzling
2 teaspoons sea salt, more for drizzling

Mixing the Batter

Whisk flour and water together in a medium bowl. Cover and let sit at room temperature for 2 to 4 hours. Batter is watery at first but will thicken with time.

Combine 2 tablespoons olive oil and salt and add to chickpea flour mixture.

Preheating the Oven and Prepping the Pan

Preheat oven to 500°F or the highest temperature your oven will go. This flatbread is traditionally made in a wood-fire oven, so a conventional oven must be extra hot.

Line a 9x13-inch baking pan with parchment paper. Grease paper surface with remaining olive oil. Alternatively, coat a well-seasoned cast iron pan with 2 tablespoons oil.

Finishing Up

Remix batter and pour it into prepared pan. Bake in preheated oven for 18 to 20 minutes or until light brown on top and edges are crisp.

Cut into individual servings and drizzle with more olive oil and sea salt. Transfer to a serving tray.

Each flatbread contains 101 calories, 6g total fat, 1g saturated fat, 0g trans fat, 0mg cholesterol, 47mg sodium, 8g carbohydrate, 1g fiber, 3g protein.

Roasted Peppers and Tomatoes
2 red peppers, cleaned and quartered
4 fresh tomatoes, sliced
2 tablespoons olive oil
1 teaspoon minced fresh herbs (flat leaf parsley, basil or oregano)
Salt and pepper
1 tablespoon capers, optional

Preheating the Oven and Prepping the Pan

Preheat oven to 350°F. Lightly grease a baking sheet or line it with parchment paper.

Baking the Peppers and Tomatoes

Brush peppers and tomatoes with olive oil, herbs, salt and pepper. Lay peppers skin side down on prepared baking sheet. Place in preheated oven and bake for 15 minutes. Turn peppers and add tomatoes to pan. Bake another 10 minutes or until peppers are easily pierced with a fork.

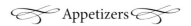
Finishing Up

Slice roasted peppers and toss with capers, if desired. Transfer tomatoes and peppers to the serving tray with the chickpea flatbread.

Artichokes

2 tablespoons olive oil
½ cup gluten-free bread crumbs
1 large egg or ¼ cup milk of choice
Salt and pepper, to taste
1 (15-ounce) can artichoke hearts, packed in water, drained and quartered
1 cup marinated olives, pitted and chopped

Getting Started

Heat olive oil in a heavy skillet.

Breading the Artichokes

Place gluten-free bread crumbs in a bowl. In a second bowl, mix together egg (or milk of choice), salt and pepper. Dip artichokes in liquid and then in bread crumbs. Add to hot oil.

Frying the Artichokes

Without stirring, cook artichokes for about 5 minutes on each side or until golden brown. Remove to a plate lined with paper towels and sprinkle with salt and pepper. Transfer to the serving tray.

To the Table

Add your favorite marinated olives, such as Kalamata, to the serving tray.

Each crostini contains 218 calories, 13g total fat, 2g saturated fat, 0g trans fat, 22mg cholesterol, 869mg sodium, 20g carbohydrate, 7g fiber, 6g protein.

> To save time, buy prepared peppers, marinated olives and artichoke hearts in oil at your local specialty store.

Chili Rellenos
Makes 6
(RECIPE BY MARY CAPONE)

Serve these smothered in chili sauce and sprinkled with fresh cheese or non-dairy cheese replacement. For best results, do not replace the eggs in this recipe.

Ingredients

6 fresh Anaheim chili peppers or 1 (7-ounce) can whole green chili peppers (fire-roasted)
½ yellow onion, chopped
2 tablespoons olive oil, for sautéing, divided
2 cloves garlic, crushed
½ teaspoon ground cumin
½ teaspoon chili powder
1 small zucchini, diced
1 (15-16 ounce) can black beans, rinsed and drained
½ cup corn, frozen, or fresh corn removed from cob
Salt and pepper, to taste
3 large eggs, separated
1 tablespoon water
3 tablespoons tapioca starch/flour
¼ teaspoon salt

Roasting the Peppers (if using fresh peppers)

If using fresh chili peppers, roast them by wiping them with olive oil and placing them on a baking pan under the broiler. Turn peppers over every few minutes until their skin is lightly blistered. When done, place in a small paper bag or bowl covered with plastic wrap to sweat and cool.

Sautéing the Vegetables

In a medium skillet, add onions to 1 tablespoon hot oil and sauté until translucent, about 3 minutes. Add garlic, cumin and chili powder and sauté for 2 minutes. Add zucchini, black beans

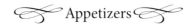

and corn and sauté until zucchini takes on color, about 5 minutes. Add salt and pepper, to taste.

Making the Egg Batter

Separate egg whites and yolks into 2 medium-size bowls. Beat whites until they form soft peaks.

Add water, tapioca starch/flour and salt to egg yolks and blend until creamy. Gently fold in egg whites to make a batter.

Stuffing the Peppers

Peel translucent skin off cooled peppers. Make a 3-inch to 4-inch slit up each pepper, keeping stem intact. Remove seeds, if desired. (Seeds increase the heat.)

Stuff peppers with equal amounts of vegetable mixture.

Finishing Up

In a heavy skillet, warm 1 tablespoon olive oil over medium heat until smoking slightly. Spoon in egg batter in the shape of a pepper. Place pepper on top of batter and cook over medium heat for 5 minutes.

Spoon more egg batter on top of pepper and then flip and cook over medium heat for another 5 minutes until golden brown. Repeat with each pepper.

Each chili contains 152 calories, 3g total fat, 1g saturated fat, 0g trans fat, 106mg cholesterol, 409mg sodium, 24g carbohydrate, 6g fiber, 9g protein.

Meatballs in Tomato Serrano Chili Sauce
Makes 18
(RECIPE BY MARY CAPONE)

These savory meatballs in spicy sauce can be served as an appetizer (offer toothpicks) or over rice as a main course.

Meatballs
2 tablespoons chopped onion
1 garlic clove, minced
2 teaspoons canned chipotle chili peppers in adobo sauce, chopped
½ pound ground beef
½ pound ground pork
½ cup gluten-free bread crumbs
1 large egg, optional
½ teaspoon Mexican oregano
1 teaspoon fresh cilantro or basil, chopped
1 teaspoon salt
Pepper, to taste

Chili Sauce
1 (28-ounce) can whole tomatoes with juice
1 teaspoon sugar
2 tablespoons cilantro, chopped
½ teaspoon dried Mexican oregano
½ teaspoon sea salt
Pepper, to taste
2 medium serrano chili peppers, roasted, stems and seeds removed
2 tablespoons olive oil
1 tablespoon butter or non-dairy alternative
2 garlic cloves, chopped

Getting Started

To make meatballs, preheat oven to 375°F. Line a baking sheet with parchment paper.

Making the Meatballs

In a medium bowl, add all meatball ingredients.

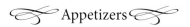
Mix together until combined. Form mixture into 1-inch meatballs and place on prepared baking sheet. Bake in preheated oven until meatballs are brown and sizzling, about 20 minutes.

Making the Sauce
To make sauce, strain tomatoes and juice through a food mill or colander to remove skin and seeds. In a medium saucepan, add tomato liquid, sugar, herbs, salt and pepper. Bring to a slow simmer, releasing water from the tomatoes and creating a paste, about 10 minutes.

Making the Chili Mixture
In a separate saucepan, add chili peppers, oil and butter. Cook over low heat until oil-butter is flavored with peppers, about 5 minutes. Add garlic and cook just until garlic begins to color, about 2 minutes. Remove peppers, tasting oil-butter sauce to check for desired flavor.

Putting It Together
Add chili mixture to tomato sauce. Add meatballs and cook to combine flavors, about 5 minutes.

Each meatball with sauce contains 107 calories, 7g total fat, 3g saturated fat, 0g trans fat, 22mg cholesterol, 292mg sodium, 6g carbohydrate, 1g fiber, 5g protein.

Multi-Color Pepper Corn Fritters
Makes 12 fritters
(RECIPE BY REBECCA REILLY)

This versatile recipe makes an appetizer that offers delicious eye appeal. Pair these colorful fritters with a spinach salad for a vegetarian lunch or serve them as a side with grilled meat. For a breakfast treat, leave out the peppers, scallions and chipotle and add a tablespoon of sugar. This recipe can be made egg-free.*

Ingredients
2 scallions, minced
¼ red pepper, seeded, chopped in ¼-inch pieces
¼ yellow pepper, seeded, chopped in ¼-inch pieces
¼ orange pepper, seeded, chopped in ¼-inch pieces
Vegetable oil or olive oil
1½ cups *Living Without's* All-Purpose Flour Blend (page xiv)
½ teaspoon salt
¾ teaspoon baking soda
⅛-¼ teaspoon ground chipotle pepper
1 large egg*
½ cup buttermilk (or ½ cup milk of choice mixed with 2 teaspoons vinegar), more to thin mixture
⅔ cup corn**
1 tablespoon olive oil
Salt, to taste

Getting Started
Sauté scallions and peppers in oil for 3 minutes. Set aside.

Making the Batter
In a medium bowl, whisk flour blend, salt, baking soda and ground chipotle together.

In a separate bowl, whisk egg and buttermilk together. Stir this into dry ingredients.

Add sautéed scallions and peppers. Add corn. If the batter seems too stiff, stir in more buttermilk.

Frying the Fritters
Heat olive oil in skillet. Drop batter teaspoon by teaspoon into hot oil. Turn once while cooking. Cook fritters until golden, about 4 minutes total.

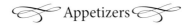
Finishing Up

Drain on paper towels. Keep warm in a low oven while continuing to cook remaining fritters. Add salt just before serving. Serve warm with Tomato Cilantro Mayonnaise.

> **Use fresh cooked corn cut from the cob or frozen corn that's thawed. To enhance the corn flavor, use grilled or roasted corn, cut from the cob.

Tomato Cilantro Mayonnaise
Makes about 1¾ cups

1 cup gluten-free, dairy-free mayonnaise
¼ cup chopped fresh cilantro leaves
½ plum tomato, seeded and finely chopped
1 small clove garlic, finely chopped
Lime juice, to taste
Salt, to taste

Putting It Together

In a bowl, gently stir together ingredients to combine. Serve with corn fritters.

Each fritter without mayonnaise contains 101 calories, 2g total fat, 0g saturated fat, 0g trans fat, 18mg cholesterol, 194mg sodium, 19g carbohydrate, 1g fiber, 1g sugars, 2g protein.

Each tablespoon of mayonnaise contains 20 calories, 1g total fat, 0g saturated fat, 0g trans fat, 0mg cholesterol, 64mg sodium, 1g carbohydrate, 0g fiber, 0g sugars, 0g protein.

> For a list of companies offering gluten-free, dairy-free, egg-free mayonnaise, see Shopping List, page 189.

> *For **Egg-Free Corn Fritters,** combine 1 tablespoon flax meal with 3 tablespoons hot water. Let sit 5 minutes until thickened. Then add to recipe.

BREADS

"There's a reason people call bread the staff of life. It's the Holy Grail for those of us who are gluten-free."

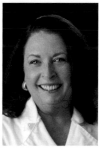

Bread recipes
by Diane Kittle
and other celebrity chefs

Diane (Dee) Kittle

Glastonbury, Connecticut

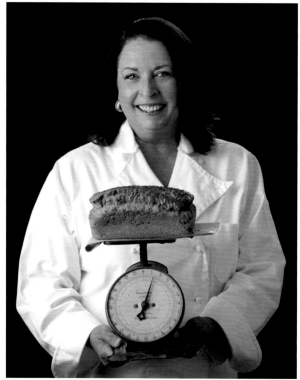

"I punch up recipes with great ingredients—organic, unrefined sugars, flavor extracts and spices."

Growing up in Maine, one of my summer "chores" was picking the bounty from my mother's enormous garden. String beans, tomatoes, raspberries, gooseberries, peppers, zucchini and more were the staples of our daily meals. My mother taught us how to make jams and pies, soups and such to highlight the fresh produce. When late summer arrived, the canning pots and jars came up from the basement to preserve the remainder of the harvest. In the winter while my father, siblings and I skied, my mother spent each Saturday cooking. Beautiful loaves of homemade bread filled the house with aromas that welcomed us home. My love of food and working with great ingredients was born from these childhood experiences.

Although I spent the first 20 years of my adult life traveling for my corporate job, each weekend was spent creating food-related memories with my family and friends—candlelit dinners, brunches and fresh baked goods.

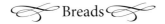

By my 40s, I was yearning for a more creative career path. I went back to school to become a pastry chef. It landed me an internship with a well-known wedding cake designer where I created artful wedding and special event cakes.

During this time, my health began to falter. I had always dealt with gastrointestinal discomfort, dairy allergies, as well as endometriosis. Now the GI issues were more acute. My doctor tested me for Lyme disease and rheumatoid arthritis with negative results. A friend suggested that I might have celiac disease. Three months later, the diagnosis was confirmed. I was delighted to know what was wrong but it meant giving up my work in the flour-filled bakery.

The day after my diagnosis, I went to the local health food store and bought a cart full of gluten-free fare—muffins, cookies, frozen breads. These goodies were too sweet, lacked flavor and had an unpleasant mouth feel.

So I started baking again, this time gluten-free. In the process of developing new recipes, I learned all about the flavor profiles and characteristics of numerous gluten-free flours, finding that many tended to lack the flavor imparted by wheat flour. I chose to punch up the flavor with great ingredients—organic, unrefined sugars, flavor extracts and spices. With experimentation, I learned how to recreate my favorite pastries and breads as gluten-free and allergy-friendly.

Over 100 recipes later, in November 2008, I opened Dee's One Smart Cookie, a bakery that is gluten free, as well as dairy, soy, peanut and tree-nut-free, with most items available egg-free as well.

I go to work each morning filled with the satisfaction of knowing we are helping many people enjoy a delicious gluten-free, allergy-friendly life.

Diane ("Dee") Kittle is an accomplished pastry chef and owner of Dee's One Smart Cookie. Located in Glastonbury, Connecticut, Dee's One Smart Cookie is the only non-GMO bakery in New England that is devoted to the production of gluten-free, dairy-free, tree nut-free, peanut-free and soy-free products.

Where to find Dee Kittle:
deesonesmartcookie.com

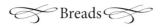

Breads

Dee's
Italian Panettone
Serves 12

One of my favorite holiday breads is panettone, studded with fruit and filled with citrus flavors. Imported from Italy and seen on the store shelves in decorative packaging during the holidays, panettone should not be confused with the much maligned fruitcake. A wonderful alternative to a sweet pastry, this bread is delicious with tea, coffee and even a dessert wine, like port. This recipe can be made egg-free.*

Ingredients
Butter or non-dairy alternative, to grease pan
Rice flour, to dust pan
2 cups rice flour (finely-ground brown rice flour works best)
⅔ cup potato starch (not potato flour)
⅓ cup tapioca starch/flour
2 teaspoons xanthan gum
1 teaspoon salt
1½ teaspoons unflavored gelatin or agar powder
¼ cup dry milk powder or non-dairy milk powder of choice
½ cup granulated sugar
1 teaspoon baking powder
1 tablespoon potato flour (not potato starch)
2¼ teaspoons (1 package) active dry yeast
2-3 teaspoons lemon zest or zest of 1 lemon
2-3 teaspoons orange zest or zest of 1 orange
½ cup golden raisins
½ cup dried cranberries
½ cup dried citron, optional**

Wet Ingredients
4 large eggs,* room temperature
2 tablespoons honey, agave nectar or maple syrup
1 teaspoon lemon extract
1 teaspoon orange extract
2 teaspoons cider vinegar
½ cup butter or non-dairy alternative, softened, or shortening
2 tablespoons gluten-free instant potato flakes
1½ cups warm orange juice (110°F–115° F)

*For **Egg-Free Panettone,** omit 4 eggs. Combine ¾ cup unsweetened applesauce with 4 teaspoons baking powder, stirring to blend. Let sit for 1 minute before adding to other wet ingredients.

Finely ground brown rice flour works best for delicate breads and cakes. To create a fine-grind flour, process regular rice flour in a clean coffee grinder until powdery.

**Citron is cubed, dried citrus fruit normally found in the dried fruit section of the grocery store, especially during the holiday season. Although this is a traditional ingredient in panettone, the use of grated zest along with raisins and dried cranberries provides a tasty alternative without the added expense.

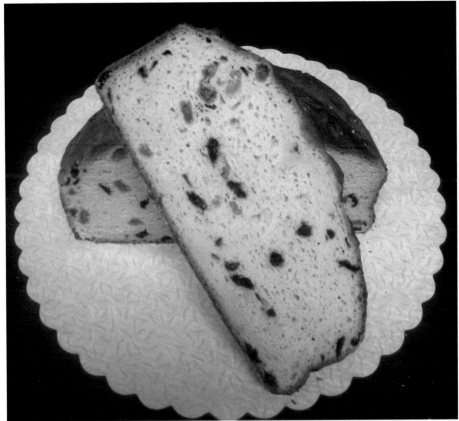

Italian Panettone

Getting Started
Grease a panettone pan or an 8-inch or 9-inch round cake pan with butter and dust with rice flour. Pat out excess flour from pan.

Mixing the Dry Ingredients
In a medium bowl, combine rice flour, potato and tapioca starches, xanthan gum, salt, gelatin, milk powder, sugar, baking powder, potato flour, yeast, lemon and orange zests, raisins, cranberries and citron, if using. Set aside.

Mixing the Wet Ingredients
In the bowl of a stand mixer fitted with the paddle attachment, place eggs, honey, lemon and orange extracts, vinegar, butter, potato flakes and orange juice and mix on medium speed for 2 minutes. Scrape down sides of mixing bowl. Don't be concerned if the butter doesn't combine completely; it will blend in once the dry ingredients are added. (Alternatively, a heavy-duty hand-held mixer can be used.)

This bread is a treat on its own but also makes superb French toast. Panettone will keep well for several days on the counter. Refrigerate after a couple of days to extend the shelf life. Toast briefly or microwave slices for 20 to 30 seconds for that "fresh from the oven" taste.

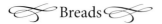
Combining Wet and Dry Mixtures
Slowly add dry ingredients to wet ingredients until blended. Scrape down sides of mixing bowl. Mix on high speed for 3 minutes. Scrape sides of bowl down again.

Letting the Dough Rise
Place the bread batter in the prepared baking pan and set in a warm place to rise for an hour. The bread will nearly double in size.

To the Oven and Out
Preheat the oven to 375°F.

Place the bread on the middle rack in the oven and bake for 50 to 60 minutes or until the internal temperature of the bread reaches 200°F to 205°F on an instant-read thermometer. Begin testing for doneness after 50 minutes.

Allow the bread to cool for 10 minutes in the pan. Tip the pan upside down on a wire rack to release the bread from the pan and cool completely.

Each serving contains 351 calories, 11g total fat, 6g saturated fat, 0g trans fat, 93mg cholesterol, 266mg sodium, 60g carbohydrate, 2g fiber, 22g sugars, 6g protein.

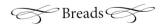

Dee's
Cardamom Bread
Serves 12

I hadn't heard of this sweet bread until a friend asked me to make it for her family's traditional Christmas celebration. This is a Scandinavian variation of Italian panettone bread. It's laced with cardamom, a flavor I adore. This recipe can be made egg-free.*

Ingredients

Butter or non-dairy alternative, to grease pan
Rice flour, to dust pan
3 cups Dee's Flour Blend #1 (page xiii)
½ cup granulated sugar
¼ cup dry milk powder or non-dairy milk powder of choice
1 tablespoon potato flour (not potato starch)
2 teaspoons xanthan gum
2 teaspoons ground cardamom
1½ teaspoons unflavored gelatin or agar powder
1 teaspoon salt
1 teaspoon baking powder
2¼ teaspoons (1 package) active dry yeast
4 large eggs,* room temperature
1½ cups warm milk of choice (110°F–115°F)
½ cup butter or non-dairy alternative, softened
2 tablespoons gluten-free instant potato flakes
2 tablespoons honey, agave nectar or pure maple syrup
2 teaspoons cider vinegar
Confectioners' sugar, for dusting, optional

Getting Started
Grease an 8-inch round cake pan with butter or non-dairy alternative and dust with rice flour. Pat out excess flour from pan.

Mixing the Dry Ingredients
Whisk together flour blend, sugar, milk powder, potato flour, xanthan gum, cardamom, gelatin, salt and baking powder in a medium bowl. Add yeast and blend. Set aside.

Mixing the Wet Ingredients
Put eggs, milk, butter, potato flakes, honey and vinegar into the large mixing bowl of a stand mixer fitted with the paddle attachment and mix

Don't have a stand mixer? This recipe can be made using a hand mixer. Just be sure to use a heavy-duty mixer.

*For **Egg-Free Cardamom Bread,** omit 4 eggs. Combine ¾ cup unsweetened applesauce with 4 teaspoons baking powder, stirring to blend. Let sit for 1 minute before adding to other wet ingredients.

When using a stand mixer, beat dough with the paddle attachment, *not* the dough hook.

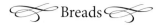

on medium speed for 2 minutes. Scrape down sides of mixing bowl. Don't be concerned if the butter doesn't combine completely; it will blend in once the dry ingredients are added.

Combining Wet and Dry Mixtures

Slowly add dry ingredients to wet ingredients until blended. Scrape down sides of mixing bowl. Mix on high speed for 3 minutes. Scrape sides of bowl down again.

Letting the Dough Rise

Using an ice cream scoop, scoop the bread batter into the prepared baking pan, placing 6 rounded scoops of batter in a circle around the bottom of the pan and 1 scoop in the center. Then repeat by adding another layer of scooped batter over the first layer. Set in a warm place to rise for 1 hour. The bread will nearly double in size.

To the Oven and Out

Preheat the oven to 375°F.

Place the bread on the middle rack in the oven and bake for approximately 60 minutes or until the internal temperature of the bread reaches 200°F to 205°F. Test for doneness after 50 minutes with an instant-read thermometer.

Allow the bread to cool for 10 minutes in the pan. Tip the pan upside down to release the bread from the pan. Once the bread cools, dust it with confectioners' sugar, if desired.

Each slice contains 314 calories, 11g total fat, 6g saturated fat, 0g trans fat, 94mg cholesterol, 277mg sodium, 49g carbohydrate, 2g fiber, 13g sugars, 6g protein.

Traditionally, cardamom bread is braided but this gluten-free dough is too loose to braid. For best results, scoop the dough into the cake pan as instructed.

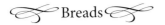
Dee's
Herby Popover Dinner Rolls
Makes 12 to 14 rolls

For many years, I lived in the Boston area and frequented a restaurant that served hot popovers instead of dinner rolls. These popovers were lightly crisp on the outside, airy on the inside, a touch custard-like on the bottom, completely irresistible…yet deceptively filling.

This recipe is a cross between those feather-light popovers and a dinner roll that is wonderfully crispy on the outside and tender on the inside. They are best served shortly after removing from the oven, which is when they are crispiest. Unlike traditional popovers, these will hold for several hours. These popover dinner rolls are yeast free.

You'll need 12 to 14 oven-safe small custard cups or a 12-vessel popover pan to make these. For best results, do not replace the eggs in this recipe.

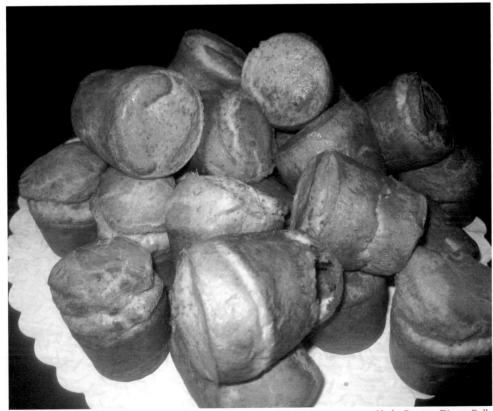

Herby Popover Dinner Rolls

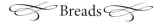

Ingredients

1½ tablespoons butter or non-dairy alternative, melted,
to grease pan or custard cups
1½ cups Dee's Flour Blend #1 (page xiii)
1 teaspoon salt
1-3 tablespoons dried dill weed or herb of choice, optional
1½ cups milk of choice, warmed or at room temperature
3 large eggs, room temperature
2 tablespoons butter or non-dairy alternative, melted

For Dinner Rolls, add ½ teaspoon xanthan gum to dry ingredients. Reduce baking time to 30 minutes. This produces a roll that is very crispy on the outside but does not rise as much during baking, making the consistency of the bread's interior more like a dinner roll.

Getting Started

Preheat oven to 400°F.

Prepping the Pan

Melt 1½ tablespoons of butter and drizzle a bit into each custard cup or popover pan. Using a pastry brush, brush the bottom and sides of the cup or pan to coat.

Place cups on a sheet pan (if using a popover pan, no sheet pan is necessary) and place in the preheated oven for 5 minutes. Heating the cups/pan before placing batter into the vessel is critical.

No peeking unless you have an oven light which allows you to see into the oven without opening the door.

Mixing the Ingredients

Meanwhile, place remaining popover ingredients into a medium mixing bowl and blend well by hand with a whisk. Place batter in a large glass measuring cup that will hold at least 4 cups.

To the Oven and Out

Once the cups/pan are pre-heated, carefully remove the sheet pan or popover pan, using oven mitts, and place on a protected surface. Fill each cup ¾ full and immediately place back in the oven. If you are using a popover pan, you will have a little batter left over. Wait for the first batch of popovers to finish baking and bake a few more with the leftover batter or prepare a few custard cups along with your popover pan and bake all at once.

Bake in preheated oven for 35 minutes. Turn onto a wire rack to cool slightly. Serve warm.

Each roll contains 106 calories, 4g total fat, 2g saturated fat, 0g trans fat, 51mg cholesterol, 193mg sodium, 16g carbohydrate, 1g fiber, 1g sugars, 2g protein.

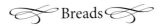

Dee's
Sticky Toffee Bread
Serves 16

Whether it's Sunday brunch or a holiday breakfast, nothing creates memories like Sticky Toffee Bread. Often referred to as "monkey" bread, this sweet, cinnamon-sugar-laced pull-apart bread is sure to get rave reviews. It's perfect with a cup of tea or coffee or as a centerpiece for your next special-occasion breakfast. Place the bread on the table warm from the oven and let your guests pull a piece and enjoy! This recipe can be made egg-free.*

Ingredients
Butter or non-dairy alternative, to grease pan
Rice flour, to dust pan
1 cup chopped pecans or walnuts, optional
4½ cups Dee's Flour Blend #3 (page xiii)
⅓ cup dry milk powder or non-dairy milk powder of choice
½ cup granulated sugar
¼ cup lightly packed brown sugar
1 tablespoon potato flour (not potato starch)
1 tablespoon xanthan gum
2 teaspoons unflavored gelatin or agar powder
1 teaspoon baking powder
1 teaspoon salt
1 tablespoon active dry yeast
5 large eggs,* room temperature
1¾ cups warm milk of choice (110°F-115°F)
½ cup butter or non-dairy alternative, softened
2 tablespoons gluten-free instant potato flakes
2 tablespoons honey, agave nectar or pure maple syrup
2 teaspoons cider vinegar

Cinnamon Sugar Coating
1¼ cups granulated sugar
1 tablespoon ground cinnamon

Sticky Toffee Topping
½ cup butter or non-dairy alternative
1 cup lightly packed brown sugar
1 tablespoon pure vanilla extract
1 pinch salt

*For **Egg-Free Sticky Toffee Bread,** omit 5 eggs. Combine ¾ cup unsweetened applesauce with 5 teaspoons baking powder, stirring to blend. Let sit for 1 minute before adding to other wet ingredients.

For dry milk powder made with potatoes, try Vance's Dari Free (vancesfoods.com). For more gluten-free, allergy-friendly products, see Shopping List, page 189.

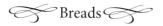

Getting Started

Grease a 10-inch bundt or tube pan with butter and dust with rice flour. Pat excess flour from pan. Do not use a removable bottom springform pan, as the topping will leak through. Place optional chopped nuts into bottom of pan and set aside.

Mixing the Dry Ingredients

Whisk together flour blend, dry milk powder, sugars, potato flour, xanthan gum, gelatin, baking powder and salt in a medium-sized bowl. Add yeast and whisk to combine. Set aside.

Mixing the Wet Ingredients

Place eggs, milk, butter, potato flakes, honey and vinegar in the large mixing bowl of a stand mixer fitted with the paddle attachment and mix on medium speed for 2 minutes. Scrape down sides of mixing bowl.

Combining Dry Ingredients with Wet Ingredients

Slowly add dry ingredients to wet ingredients until blended. Scrape down sides of mixing bowl. Mix on high speed for 4 minutes. Scrape sides of bowl down again. The dough should be similar in consistency to a thick cake batter.

Making the Sugar Coating

In a bowl, blend the granulated sugar and cinnamon together for the Cinnamon Sugar Coating.

Scooping the Dough into the Pan

With a small scoop (such as a 1-inch cookie dough scoop), drop the dough into the Cinnamon Sugar Coating. Using scoop, gently roll dough to cover it with the Cinnamon Sugar Coating. Then scoop the dough back into the scoop and drop into the prepared bundt pan. Continue this process, gently dropping the cinnamon sugar dough balls into the pan so they overlap, until all the dough is used and the pan is approximately ⅔ to ¾ full.

Making the Sticky Toffee Topping

Place the Sticky Toffee Topping ingredients into a medium saucepan and set over medium heat. Allow the ingredients to melt and then come to a slight boil, approximately 5 minutes, stirring occasionally. Using a large spoon, gently pour the liquid over the top of the dough.

Letting the Dough Rise

Place the bread pan in a warm place and let it rise for an hour. The bread

Don't have a stand mixer? This recipe can be made using a heavy-duty hand mixer.

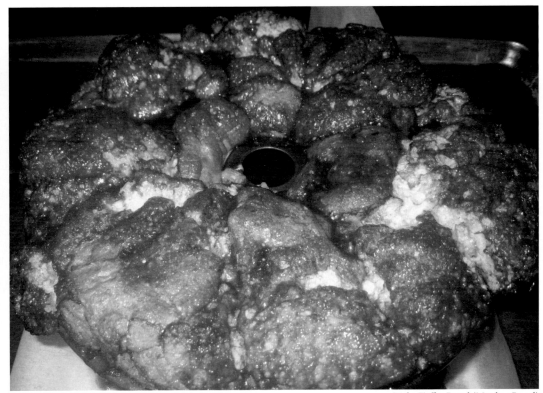
Sticky Toffee Bread (Monkey Bread)

should rise to nearly the top of the pan. Preheat the oven to 375°F.

To the Oven and Out

Cover a baking sheet or cookie pan with parchment paper. Place the bread pan on the covered sheet pan and place in preheated oven. Some of the topping will ooze over the sides during the baking process as the bread will continue to rise during baking. Bake for 50 to 60 minutes, checking the internal temperature of the bread after 50 minutes. The bread is done when the internal temperature reaches 205°F to 210°F.

Allow the bread to cool for 5 to 10 minutes in the pan. Place a serving dish upside down on the top of the pan. Then quickly invert the bread onto the serving dish, wearing oven mitts to prevent burns. The bread should release from the pan, though a little coaxing around the sides of the pan with a flat knife might be necessary. Pull the pan up and off the bread. The sticky topping will ooze down onto the bread. If there are nuts or any additional topping left in the pan, use a spoon to place them on the top of the bread. Let cool for an additional 10 minutes before serving.

Each slice serving contains 475 calories, 30g total fat, 9g saturated fat, 0g trans fat, 100mg cholesterol, 96mg sodium, 84g carbohydrate, 2g fiber, 42g sugars, 5g protein.

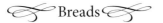

Dee's
Champion Sandwich Bread
Makes 2 loaves

Light in texture, this is the perfect everyday bread for breakfast and sandwiches. This recipe takes only a few minutes to put together in a stand mixer. For maximum yeast rise, have all ingredients at room temperature. This recipe can be made egg-free.*

Ingredients
4 cups Dee's Flour Blend #2 (page xiii)
1 tablespoon xanthan gum
1 tablespoon gluten-free egg replacer**
2 teaspoons salt
½ cup dry milk powder or non-dairy milk powder of choice
2¼ teaspoons (1 package) active dry yeast
3 large eggs,* room temperature
¼ cup butter, non-dairy alternative or shortening
2 teaspoons cider vinegar
⅓ cup honey or agave nectar
2 cups warm water (110°F-115°F)

Getting Started
Grease and flour two 8x4-inch bread pans.

Mixing the Dry Ingredients
Mix dry ingredients together in a medium-size bowl. Set aside.

Mixing the Wet Ingredients
Place eggs, butter, vinegar and honey in the mixing bowl of a stand mixer. With the paddle attachment, mix ingredients together for about 30 seconds. The butter will be chunky.

Combining the Mixtures (Wet and Dry)
Add half the dry ingredients to the wet mixture. Mix just until blended. Add remaining dry ingredients and mix for approximately 30 seconds until blended.

With the mixer on low speed, slowly add warm water until well absorbed. Turn the mixer to medium-high speed and beat for 4 minutes. Bread dough should resemble cake batter.

*For **Egg-Free Champion Sandwich Bread,** omit 3 eggs. Combine 9 tablespoons unsweetened applesauce with 3 teaspoons baking powder, stirring to blend. Let sit for 1 minute before adding to other wet ingredients.

**Gluten-free egg replacer is available from Ener-G Foods (ener-g.com).

For **Sesame Bread,** add 1 tablespoon sesame seeds to the batter after dough has mixed for 4 minutes. Then blend an additional 30 seconds. Spoon dough into prepared pans. With a pastry brush, brush the top of each loaf with a beaten egg white or milk of choice and sprinkle with additional sesame seeds. Spoon batter into loaf pans and bake as directed.

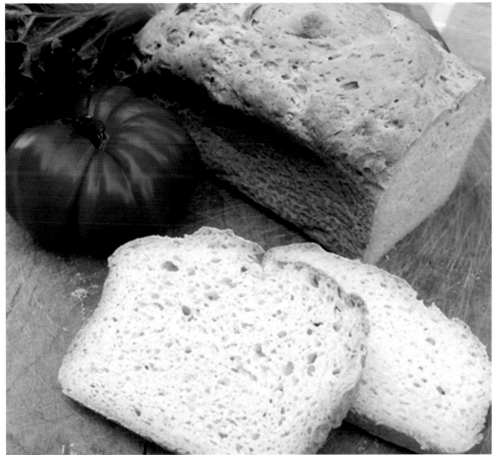

Champion Sandwich Bread

To the Oven and Out

Spoon the dough into prepared pans. Set aside in a warm place to rise, about 50 to 60 minutes. While dough rises, preheat oven to 375°F.

Place pans in preheated oven on middle rack and bake for 50 to 60 minutes or until bread's internal temperature reaches 200°F with an instant-read thermometer.

Let bread cool in pans for 10 minutes. Then remove loaves from pans and place on a rack to cool.

For **Granola Bread,** add 1½ cups seeds, dried fruit and/or nuts (if tolerated) to the batter after the dough has been mixed for 4 minutes. Blend an additional minute to combine. Spoon batter into loaf pans and bake as directed.

Each serving contains 119 calories, 3g total fat, 2g saturated fat, 0g trans fat, 29mg cholesterol, 185mg sodium, 21g carbohydrate, 1g fiber, 0g protein.

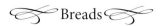

Dee's
Oatmeal Maple Bread
Makes 2 loaves

No kneading. No proofing the yeast. No problem! This bread has great texture, perfect for sandwiches or toast. The maple syrup does double duty, adding flavor and activating the yeast. This recipe makes delicious rolls with a thick, crispy crust and an airy, slightly chewy interior. It can be made egg-free.*

Ingredients
Butter or non-dairy alternative, to grease pan
Brown rice flour, to dust pan
2 cups brown rice flour, preferably super-fine grind
1 cup gluten-free oat flour
1½ cups sorghum flour or millet flour
1 cup tapioca starch/flour
½ cup potato starch (not flour)
½ cup sweet rice flour
4½ teaspoons (2 packages) active dry yeast
1 tablespoon + 1 teaspoon xanthan gum
1 tablespoon salt
5 large eggs,* room temperature
4 tablespoons pure maple syrup or amber agave nectar
½ cup shortening, butter or non-dairy alternative, melted
2½ cups warm milk of choice (110°F to 115°F)
1 egg white,* lightly beaten with a fork, to brush tops of loaves
½ cup gluten-free oats

Getting Started
Prepare two 9x5-inch bread pans (or two 8x4-inch bread pans and 6 muffin tins) by greasing well and dusting with brown rice flour. Set aside.

Mixing the Ingredients
Place brown rice flour, oat flour, sorghum flour, tapioca starch/flour, potato starch, sweet rice flour, dry yeast, xanthan gum and salt into the mixing bowl of a stand mixer with a paddle attachment. Mix on low speed for a few seconds just to combine ingredients.

In separate bowl, hand whisk the eggs, maple syrup, shortening and milk. Add the wet ingredients to the dry ingredients and mix until combined. Then mix for 5 minutes on medium-high speed. Batter will resemble a very thick cake batter.

No oat flour? Make it by processing gluten-free oats in a food processor with the steel blade attachment for 1 minute.

Super-fine rice flour ensures a smooth-textured loaf. To make it, process regular rice flour in a clean coffee grinder or a food processor with the steel blade attachment until powdery.

*For **Egg-Free Oatmeal Maple Bread,** omit 5 eggs. Combine 1 cup unsweetened applesauce with 5 teaspoons baking powder, stirring to blend. Let sit for 1 minute before adding to the remaining wet ingredients. Lightly brush unbaked bread or rolls with 1 tablespoon milk of choice; then sprinkle gluten-free oats on top.

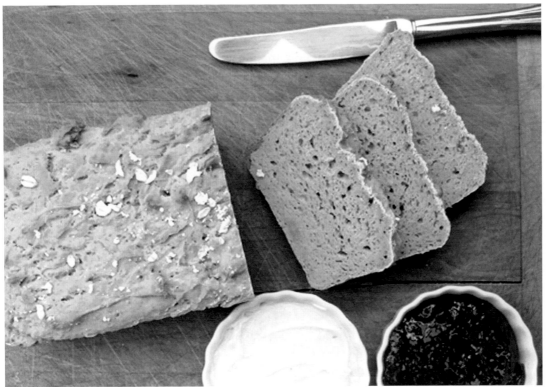

Oatmeal Maple Bread

To the Oven and Out

Spoon batter into prepared pans. This recipe makes two 9-inch loaves or two 8-inch loaves plus 6 dinner rolls. To make the rolls, use a large ice cream scoop to portion the batter into 6 standard-size muffin cups; then divide remaining batter into two 8-inch bread pans.

Using a pastry brush, lightly brush the top of the dough with egg white or non-dairy milk of choice. Sprinkle gluten-free oats on top.

Let dough rise in a warm place for approximately 40 minutes or until nearly doubled in size. Preheat oven to 350°F.

Place bread pans in preheated oven and bake for approximately 30 (for rolls) to 40 minutes (for loaves). Bread is done when internal temperature reads 200°F on an instant-read thermometer.

Cool bread in pans for 10 minutes. Remove from pans and cool on a rack.

Each serving contains 150 calories, 5g total fat, 2g saturated fat, 0g trans fat, 35mg cholesterol, 231mg sodium, 24g carbohydrate, 1g fiber, 3g protein.

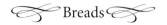

Mock Rye Bread
Makes 2 loaves
(RECIPE BY DIANE KITTLE)

There's no rye in this bread but you'll be taken by the rye-bread flavor and texture. This recipe can be made egg-free.*

Ingredients

4 cups *Living Without's* High-Protein Flour Blend (page xiv)
1 tablespoon xanthan gum
2 teaspoons salt
½ cup almond meal, dry milk powder or non-dairy milk powder of choice
2 tablespoons caraway seeds, more for sprinkling on top
1 tablespoon unsweetened cocoa powder
2¼ teaspoons (1 package) active dry yeast
1 teaspoon rye flavor powder, optional
2 large eggs,* room temperature
1 egg white*
1 teaspoon cider vinegar
¼ cup shortening or non-dairy butter alternative
1 tablespoon organic molasses or unsulphured molasses
4 tablespoons agave nectar or brown sugar
1 teaspoon coffee extract or
1 tablespoon instant coffee granules
2 cups warm milk of choice or water (110°F -115°F)

Getting Started
Grease two 8x4-inch loaf pans or two 8-inch round cake pans (at least 2 inches deep) and dust with rice flour.

Mixing the Ingredients
In a medium bowl, combine flour blend, xanthan gum, salt, almond meal or dry milk powder, cocoa powder, dry yeast and rye flavor powder, if desired. Set aside.

In mixing bowl of a stand mixer, combine eggs, egg white, cider vinegar, shortening, molasses, agave nectar and coffee extract. Mix ingredients together on medium-low speed for 1 minute to blend. Shortening will be lumpy.

Add milk or water to the wet ingredients and mix on low for 30 seconds.

Add half the dry ingredients to the wet ingredients and mix until just blended. Add remaining dry ingredients and blend. Then beat at medium-high speed for 4 minutes.

To the Oven and Out
Spoon batter into prepared pans and set in a warm place to rise, about 50 minutes or until doubled in size. Preheat oven to 375°F.

Bake in preheated oven for approximately 50 minutes until done. Bread is done when internal temperature reads 200°F on an instant-read thermometer. Bread may darken quickly. If so, tent loaves with aluminum foil while baking.

Each serving contains 106 calories, 3g total fat, 0g saturated fat, 0g trans fat, 15mg cholesterol, 208mg sodium, 18g carbohydrate, 1g fiber, 2g protein.

*For **Egg-Free Mock Rye Bread,** omit 2 eggs and 1 egg white. Combine 6 tablespoons unsweetened applesauce with 2 teaspoons baking powder, stirring to blend. Let sit for 1 minute. Combine 1 tablespoon flax meal with 2 tablespoons warm water. Let sit for 5 minutes until slightly thickened. Add applesauce mixture and flax meal mixture to the wet ingredients.

Gluten-free rye flavor powder is available from Authentic Foods (authenticfoods.com).

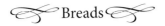

Tropical Bread
Makes 2 loaves
(RECIPE BY DIANE KITTLE)

This high-protein bread has a springy texture that's great toasted and makes scrumptious French toast. The natural sugars in the crushed pineapple and orange juice cause this bread to brown quickly. To prevent over-browning, loosely cover loaves with aluminum foil 10 minutes after bread begins baking. This recipe can be made egg-free.*

Ingredients
4½ cups *Living Without's* High-Protein Flour Blend (page xiv)
1 tablespoon xanthan gum
1 teaspoon baking soda
1 teaspoon salt
¼ cup almond meal, dry milk powder or non-dairy milk powder of choice
3 large eggs,* room temperature
1 teaspoon cider vinegar
4 tablespoons agave nectar
⅓ cup shortening or non-dairy butter alternative, room temperature
2 (6-ounce) cans crushed pineapple with juice
½ cup warm orange juice (110°F)
1 tablespoon + 1 teaspoon active dry yeast

Getting Started
Grease and flour two 8x4-inch loaf pans.

Mixing the Ingredients
In a medium-size bowl, combine flour blend, xanthan gum, baking soda, salt, almond meal or milk powder and set aside.

In the mixing bowl of a stand mixer with paddle attachment, combine eggs, cider vinegar, agave nectar, shortening and crushed pineapple with juice. Mix on low speed until combined. Shortening will be lumpy.

In a small bowl, stir yeast into orange juice and let sit to proof about 10 minutes. Yeast mixture will double in size. Set aside.

Add dry ingredients to egg mixture and mix for approximately 1 minute until well combined. Add yeast mixture and mix on low speed for 30 seconds. Then increase speed to medium-high and beat for 4 minutes.

To the Oven and Out
Spoon batter into prepared pans and let rise in a warm place for approximately 45 minutes or until nearly doubled in size. While bread is rising, preheat oven to 350°F.

Place bread in oven and bake for approximately 50 minutes until done. Bread is done when internal temperature reads 200°F on an instant-read thermometer.

Each serving contains 72 calories, 3g total fat, 1g saturated fat, 0g trans fat, 24mg cholesterol, 223mg sodium, 10g carbohydrate, 0g fiber, 2g protein.

*For **Egg-Free Tropical Bread,** omit 3 eggs. Combine 9 tablespoons unsweetened applesauce with 3 teaspoons baking powder, stirring to blend. Let sit for 1 minute before adding to other wet ingredients.

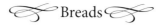

Baguettes
Makes 2 baguettes
(RECIPE BY REBECCA REILLY)

This recipe makes marvelous gluten-free bread in just 2 hours. Slice and feast! Use baguettes for garlic bread, crostini, submarine sandwiches, baguette pizza and even French toast. This recipe can be made egg-free.*

Ingredients
3 cups *Living Without's* High-Protein Flour Blend (page xiv)
1 tablespoon cornmeal, more for dusting
2 teaspoons sugar of choice
1 tablespoon xanthan gum
4½ teaspoons (2 packages) rapid rise yeast
¾ teaspoon salt
1¼ cups warm water (110°F-115°F)
1 teaspoon cider vinegar
2 large eggs,* room temperature
3 tablespoons extra-virgin olive oil

Getting Started
Line a double baguette form with foil, extending foil up the sides by 2 inches. Lightly grease foil and sprinkle with cornmeal. Alternatively, make 2 baguette-shaped forms (each measuring 2 inches wide, 4 inches high, 14 to 16 inches long) using a double thickness of heavy-duty foil, dull side out; lightly grease and sprinkle each with gluten-free flour or cornmeal and place on a cookie sheet.

Making the Dough
Mix dry ingredients together in the bowl of a stand mixer.

In a separate bowl, whisk together the water, vinegar, eggs and oil. Add to dry ingredients. Using the beater or paddle of your mixer (not the whisk), beat mixture on low speed until well

blended. Then turn the speed up and beat for 5 minutes on medium-high speed.

Forming the Baguettes
With oiled hands or oiled plastic wrap, divide dough in half and shape into 2 baguettes. Place in prepared pan and cover with lightly greased plastic wrap. Let rise in a warm place for 20 to 30 minutes.

To the Oven and Out
Preheat oven to 375°F. Spritz dough with water. Place in preheated oven and bake for 30 minutes or until done. Bread is done when internal temperature reaches 200°F.

Each serving contains 154 calories, 4g total fat, 1g saturated fat, 0g trans fat, 40mg cholesterol, 128mg sodium, 26g carbohydrate, 1g fiber, 4g protein.

*For **Egg-Free Baguettes,** omit 2 eggs. Combine 6 tablespoons unsweetened applesauce with 2 teaspoons baking powder, stirring to blend. Let sit for 1 minute before adding to other wet ingredients.

Brioche Bread
Serves 6 to 8
(RECIPE BY REBECCA REILLY)

This versatile French yeast bread can be enjoyed for breakfast or stuffed with a savory filling and served with salad for dinner. Slice it for French toast or toast it and top it with non-dairy ice cream and fresh berries for dessert. This recipe can be made egg-free.*

Ingredients
3 cups *Living Without's* High-Protein Flour Blend (page xiv)
1 tablespoon xanthan gum
½ teaspoon salt

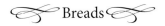

6 tablespoons sugar
4½ teaspoons (2 packages) rapid rise yeast
1 teaspoon cider vinegar
3 large eggs,* room temperature
1 cup milk of choice, tepid, divided
12 tablespoons (1½ sticks) unsalted butter, softened, or non-dairy alternative
Zest of 1 lemon, optional

Getting Started
Grease a brioche mold or medium bundt pan.

Making the Dough
Mix flour, xanthan gum, salt, sugar and yeast together in the bowl of a heavy-duty mixer.

Using the paddle of the mixer on medium speed, blend in vinegar, eggs and ½ cup milk. Add remaining ½ cup milk and scrape the sides. Beat in soft butter, tablespoon by tablespoon. Then beat for 3 minutes. Add lemon zest, if desired.

Finishing Up
Using an ice cream scoop, scoop the dough evenly into the prepared mold or bundt pan. Cover with lightly oiled plastic wrap and set in a warm place to rise for 20 to 30 minutes.

To the Oven and Out
Preheat oven to 375°F. Place pan in oven and bake for 20 minutes. Then lower heat to 350°F and bake another 20 minutes or until internal temperature reaches 200°F. If bread browns too quickly, cover loosely with foil for the second half of baking.

Each serving contains 400 calories, 21g total fat, 7g saturated fat, 0g trans fat, 101mg cholesterol, 199mg sodium, 47g carbohydrate, 2g fiber, 7g protein.

*For **Egg-Free Brioche Bread,** omit 3 eggs. Add 1 tablespoon arrowroot to the dry ingredients.

Combine 2 tablespoons flax meal with 6 tablespoons warm water. Let sit for 5 minutes until slightly thickened before adding to other wet ingredients. If bread browns too quickly, cover the loaf loosely with foil during last 15 minutes of baking time.

Egg Bread
Makes 1 loaf
(RECIPE BY REBECCA REILLY)

Egg yolks and bean flour give this soft-textured bread a light golden color. This recipe makes delicious sandwich bread, rolls and baguettes. It can be made egg-free.*

Ingredients
3 cups *Living Without's* High-Protein Flour Blend (page xiv)
¼ cup dry milk powder of choice
1 tablespoon xanthan gum
1 teaspoon salt
4½ teaspoons (2 packages) instant dry yeast
3 large eggs,* room temperature
1 teaspoon cider vinegar
¼ cup melted butter or extra virgin olive oil
1 tablespoon honey or agave nectar
1 cup warm water (110°F-115°F)

Getting Started
Lightly grease a 9x4-inch bread pan and sprinkle with cornmeal or rice flour.

Making the Dough
Mix flour blend, milk powder, xanthan gum and salt in a mixing bowl until well blended. Using the beater/paddle, mix in the yeast.

Whisk eggs, vinegar, melted butter, honey and warm water together.

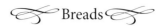
Pour wet ingredients into the dry, mixing on medium speed until everything is well blended. If the batter seems too dry, add more water, 1 tablespoon at a time. Beat on medium-high speed for 5 minutes.

Finishing Up

Spoon the dough into the prepared pan. Spray the top of the dough with baking spray. Use the back of a spoon to smooth the top. Spray a piece of plastic wrap and loosely cover the bread. Place in a warm, draft-free place for 30 minutes or until the dough reaches a ¼ inch from the top of the pan.

To the Oven and Out

Preheat oven to 375°F. Place pan in oven on the middle rack and bake 35 to 45 minutes until done. Remove from the pan and cool on a rack.

Each slice contains 138 calories, 5g total fat, 2g saturated fat, 0g trans fat, 49mg cholesterol, 171mg sodium, 20g carbohydrate, 1g fiber, 2g sugars, 4g protein.

> *For **Egg-Free Egg Bread,** omit 3 eggs. Add 2 teaspoons of baking powder to dry ingredients. Combine 1 tablespoon flax meal with 3 tablespoons warm water. Let sit for 5 minutes until slightly thickened. Add 6 tablespoons unsweetened applesauce to flax mixture and combine with wet ingredients.
>
> For a slightly crisper crust, add 2 tablespoons cornmeal to the dry ingredients and omit the powdered milk.
>
> For 2 **Egg Bread Baguettes,** use a double baguette pan, lined with a double thickness of foil (dull side out), lightly oiled and generously sprinkled with cornmeal or rice flour. Make sure the foil is about 3 inches higher than the sides of the pan. Spoon half the batter into each channel. Smooth the tops with the back of an oiled soup spoon. Place dough in a warm, draft-free spot. Loosely cover with lightly oiled plastic wrap. Let the dough rise to the rim of the baguette pans. Bake in preheated 375°F

oven for 25 minutes. Then slide the loaves out of the pan and continue baking on the middle oven rack for another 5 minutes. Remove from oven and cool on a rack.

For **Egg Bread Rolls,** spray a muffin tin and dust with cornmeal or rice flour. Fill each cup halfway with dough and loosely cover with oiled plastic wrap. Let dough rise to the top of pan. Bake in preheated 375°F oven for 25 minutes or until done.

Hawaiian Sweet Bread
Makes one loaf
(RECIPE BY MARY CAPONE)

Similar to Portuguese sweet bread or pao doce, this bread has a rich texture and slightly sweet taste. This bread makes delicious French toast. It can be made egg-free.* Makes one 9x5-inch loaf or two 6-inch round boules.

Ingredients
½ cup warm water (110°F-115°F)
2 teaspoons sugar
4½ teaspoons (2 packages) active dry yeast
2 cups brown rice flour
½ cup potato starch (not potato flour)
½ cup tapioca starch/flour
½ cup sugar
1 tablespoon xanthan gum
1 teaspoon salt
3 tablespoons vegetable oil or melted butter
3 large eggs*
½ cup warm milk of choice (110°F-115°F)

Getting Started

Lightly grease a 9x5-inch loaf pan or two 6-inch round cake pans.

Mixing the Ingredients

In a small bowl, combine warm water, 2 teaspoons sugar and yeast. Stir just until dissolved. Cover

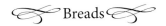

with a clean kitchen towel and set aside in a warm area for 10 minutes. Mixture will form a foam head about an inch tall.**

Place rice flour, potato starch, tapioca starch/flour, ½ cup sugar, xanthan gum and salt in the bowl of a food processor or heavy-duty stand mixer with paddle attachment. Blend dry ingredients together, until well combined. If mixing by hand, place dry ingredients in a large mixing bowl and whisk together until well combined.

In a small bowl, whisk oil or melted butter, eggs and warm milk until blended.

Add egg mixture to dry ingredients and combine. Add yeast mixture to dough and mix again until dough forms. If mixing with a heavy-duty stand mixer, this process takes about 5 minutes. With a food processor, about 2 to 3 minutes. By hand, about 10 minutes. Dough will be soft and sticky.

To the Oven and Out
Transfer dough into prepared pan(s). Smooth top into desired shape with wet hands or a spatula dipped in water. Place in a warm area to rise for 40 minutes.

Score loaf top about ¼-inch deep with a sharp knife. If a shiny surface is desired, brush with an egg mixed with 1 tablespoon water (or brush with milk of choice).

Preheat oven to 350°F. Place pan(s) in oven and bake for 40 to 45 minutes for a loaf, 35 to 40 minutes for two boules. Bread is done when bottom sounds hollow when tapped and internal temperature reaches 195°F to 200°F.

Each slice contains 168 calories, 4g total fat, 1g saturated fat, 0g trans fat, 40mg cholesterol, 164mg sodium, 30g carbohydrate, 1g fiber, 3g protein.

*For **Egg-Free Hawaiian Sweet Bread**, omit 3 eggs. Combine 2 tablespoons flax meal with 6 tablespoons warm water. Let sit for 5 minutes until slightly thickened. Combine 1½ teaspoons Ener-G egg replacer powder with 2 teaspoons warm water. Then add flax meal mixture and egg replacer mixture to wet ingredients.

**If yeast mixture does not foam, either the yeast is not viable or your water is too hot or cold. Throw out the yeast mixture and start again with fresh yeast.

Herb and Garlic Breadsticks
Makes 18
(RECIPE BY MARY CAPONE)

These breadsticks are family favorites and can be prepared quickly. This recipe can be made egg-free.*

Ingredients
½ cup water
¼ cup olive oil
¾ teaspoon salt
Dash pepper
1 pinch freshly grated nutmeg
½ cup Mary's All-Purpose Flour Blend
(page xiv)
1 teaspoon xanthan gum
2 large eggs*
1 tablespoon fresh herbs (thyme, parsley, basil), chopped
1 clove garlic, minced, optional

Getting Started
Preheat oven to 425°F. Lightly grease 2 baking sheets or line them with parchment paper.

Making the Dough
In a medium saucepan, heat water, oil, salt, pepper and nutmeg over medium heat until liquid

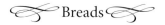

begins to simmer. Mix flour blend with xanthan gum and immediately add to saucepan, stirring until dough forms. Cook for 2 minutes over low heat, stirring constantly.

Pour the hot mixture into a food processor. Add eggs, herbs and garlic, if desired, and pulse until ingredients are incorporated and dough is smooth and elastic.

Forming the Breadsticks
Spoon mixture into a pastry bag. A #14 bag with the coupling attached and no tip is just the right size for breadsticks. If you don't have a pastry bag, use a large zip-top plastic bag with about ½-inch of a corner trimmed off. Squeeze out long, thin mounds of dough (8 to 10 inches long, ½ inch wide) onto prepared baking sheets. Use wet fingers to lightly press down the ends.

To the Oven and Out
Bake breadsticks in preheated oven until golden brown, about 20 to 24 minutes.

Each breadstick contains 51 calories, 4g total fat, 1g saturated fat, 0g trans fat, 23mg cholesterol, 105mg sodium, 4g carbohydrate, 0g fiber, 1g protein.

*For **Egg-Free Herb and Garlic Breadsticks**, omit 2 eggs. Add 1 tablespoon arrowroot to flour blend and xanthan gum and mix well. Combine 1 tablespoon flax meal with 3 tablespoons warm water. Let sit for 5 minutes until slightly thickened. Add flax meal mixture to wet ingredients in the saucepan, mixing well before adding the dry ingredients.

Masterful Pizza Crust
Makes 2 12-inch crusts
(RECIPE BY BETH HILLSON)

Use this recipe as the base for Gourmet Pizza or top this crust with your favorite topping. Either way, this recipe is sure to become a family staple. No need to let the dough rise; it puffs up nicely in the oven. This recipe is egg-free.

Ingredients
2½ cups *Living Without's* High-Protein Flour Blend (page xiv)
½ cup millet flour
1 tablespoon xanthan gum
1 teaspoon salt
2 teaspoons chopped dry or 1 tablespoon chopped fresh rosemary, optional
5 teaspoons instant dry yeast
1⅓ cups warm water (110°F-115°F)
2 tablespoons olive oil
1 tablespoon honey
1 teaspoon cider vinegar

Making the Dough
In the bowl of a heavy-duty mixer fitted with the paddle attachment, combine the high-protein blend, millet flour, xanthan gum, salt and rosemary, if used. Blend well. Add the yeast and blend.

In a small bowl, combine water, oil, honey and vinegar. Add to dry ingredients. Beat at medium-high speed for 3 to 5 minutes or until the dough thickens.

Preparing the Crust
Scoop half the dough onto a lightly oiled sheet of parchment paper. Cover with lightly oiled plastic wrap. Use fingertips and palm to lightly press the dough into a 12-inch circle. Then form a rim of dough around the edge. Repeat

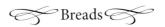

with remaining dough to make a second crust. Remove plastic wrap before adding toppings.

There's no need to let this dough rise before baking. However, if you like a thicker crust, let the dough rise for 10 minutes before adding toppings.

Gourmet Pizza
Makes 2 12-inch pizzas

1 recipe Master Pizza Dough
4 teaspoons olive oil, divided
4 tablespoons pizza sauce, divided
6 medium tomatoes (red, yellow and orange), thickly sliced
2 handfuls small, pitted, cured black olives, such as Nicoise
½ cup cubed Manchego or dairy-free cheese, divided, optional
Freshly grated Parmesan cheese or non-dairy alternative
Fresh rosemary, for garnish

Preheating the Oven
Preheat oven to 450°F. If using a pizza stone, place it on the lowest rack before preheating the oven. Do this 30 to 60 minutes ahead so the stone is very hot. If you're not using a stone, it's not necessary to preheat the oven for an extended period of time.

Topping the Pizza
Drizzle half the olive oil over the surface of 1 pizza crust. Top with 2 tablespoons pizza sauce, spreading sauce evenly over surface.

Scatter half the tomato slices, olives and cheese over the sauce. Sprinkle with freshly grated Parmesan.

To the Oven and Out
Slide pizza (with parchment paper) onto a pizza paddle and transfer to preheated stone, sliding pizza and parchment off the paddle and onto the stone. If using a baking sheet, slide pizza and parchment onto a baking sheet and set it on the lowest rack of preheated oven. Bake 18 to 22 minutes. (If crust is thicker, bake an additional 3 to 4 minutes.)

When done, the bottom of the pizza will be brown. (While first pizza is baking, repeat with remaining dough and ingredients.)

Slide pizza paddle under the parchment and slide the pizzas out of the oven. (Don't worry if the paper tears a little.) Sprinkle pizzas with fresh rosemary and serve warm.

Each slice contains 110 calories, 4g total fat, 1g saturated fat, 0g trans fat, 4mg cholesterol, 183mg sodium, 53g carbohydrate, 4g fiber, 15g protein.

Stuffing Rolls
Makes 24 rolls
(RECIPE BY BETH HILLSON)

Here's a way to serve both bread and stuffing, all rolled into one. This portable item can be served for buffet or potluck and also works beautifully for a formal sit-down meal. To reheat, place rolls in preheated 350°F oven for 5 minutes. This recipe can be made egg-free.*

Stuffing
2 tablespoons olive oil, divided
2 large uncooked gluten-free chicken-apple sausages, casing removed (½–¾ pound)
1 medium onion, diced
1 large apple, peeled and diced
3 teaspoons poultry seasoning, to taste

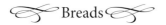

Dough

4 cups *Living Without's* High-Protein Flour
Blend (page xiv)
4 teaspoons xanthan gum
1½ teaspoons salt
2 tablespoons sugar
3 teaspoons active dry yeast
1½ cups warm milk of choice (105°F-115°F)
3 large eggs*
4 tablespoons melted butter or oil of choice

Making the Stuffing Mixture

Heat 1 tablespoon olive oil in a medium skillet.
Crumble sausage and sauté until slightly
brown. Add remaining olive oil, onion and
apple. Cook mixture until onion and apple
are soft and sausage is cooked through. Stir
in poultry seasoning, to taste. Remove from
heat and allow to cool to room temperature.
Chop sausage mixture with the back of a spoon
or on a cutting board. Measure out about 2½
cups. Reserve. (Set aside any extra stuffing for
another use.)

Getting Started

Coat 24 muffin cups with vegetable spray. Set
aside.

Making the Dough

In a large mixing bowl, combine flour blend,
xanthan gum, salt and sugar. Mix well. Stir in
yeast to combine.

In a separate bowl, combine milk, eggs and
melted butter or oil, mixing well. Add to dry
ingredients. Beat on low speed until combined.

Then beat on medium-high for 3 minutes.
Fold in reserved 2½ cups chopped stuffing
mixture.

Finishing Up

Scoop into prepared muffin tins. Cover with
lightly oiled plastic wrap and set in a warm
place to rise until doubled in size, about 30 to 40
minutes.

Preheat oven to 350°F.

To the Oven and Out

Remove plastic wrap. Place rolls in preheated
oven and bake 22 to 25 minutes. When done, remove from oven and cool to room temperature.

Each roll contains 148 calories, 6g total fat,1g saturated
fat, 0g trans fat, 36mg cholesterol, 237mg sodium, 20g
carbohydrate, 1g fiber, 4g protein.

*For **Egg-Free Stuffing Rolls,** omit 3 eggs.
Combine 3 tablespoons flax meal with 9
tablespoons warm milk of choice. Let sit for 5
minutes until slightly thickened. Add flax meal
mixture to other wet ingredients. If dough seems
too dry, slowly add more milk, 1 teaspoon at
time. Egg-free rolls may bake more quickly.
Begin checking after 20 minutes in the oven.

SOUPS

"Soup is a superfood that multitasks."

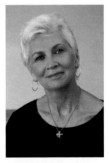

Recipes by
Sueson Vess
and other celebrity chefs

Sueson Vess

Pinehurst, North Carolina

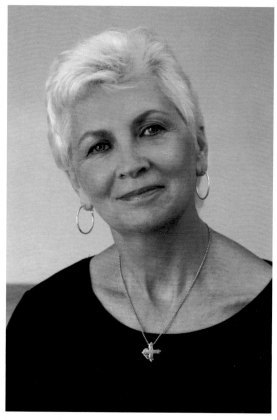

"Everything we eat has the power to build up or tear down our health."

I love great-tasting food. I'm a foodie and have always enjoyed cooking and experimenting in the kitchen. Healthy gluten-free, allergy-friendly living is my passion. But it wasn't always that way. As the mother of four boys, I spent a lot of time cooking meals my family would enjoy, but they weren't necessarily nutritious. At the time, I was unaware of beneficial and harmful foods.

My eyes were opened in 2001 when I was diagnosed with celiac disease and multiple food intolerances and I had to say good-bye to gluten, dairy and sugar. Although my new diet was a challenge, my renewed energy and restored health inspired me to find and make foods that were not only safe, but also packed the most nutrition into every bite and still tasted good.

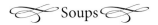

"Foods with benefits" became my mantra. Helping others on a similar journey became my mission.

All of this prompted my enormous appreciation for soup. It is a superfood that multitasks.

Soups, sauces, salsas and smoothies share more than the letter "S." A favorite marinara sauce over pasta can transform into tomato soup with the addition of a flavorful broth. Even store-bought Mexican salsa can be converted into chicken tortilla soup with the addition of broth, leftover chicken and cut-up gluten-free tortillas. Transforming a cantaloupe or peach smoothie into a cool and refreshing gazpacho is as easy as adding broth and seasonings.

Make every bite count. Stay away from empty calories. Pack the nutrition into what you do eat. And explore, experiment and have fun on your journey to better health.

Sueson Vess is a chef, food writer and educator who specializes in helping those with celiac disease, food intolerances, autism and chronic illnesses. She focuses on "foods with benefits," replacing gluten and dairy with delicious and nutritious foods that love you back.

Vess is author of *Special Eats: Simple, Delicious Solutions for Gluten & Dairy Free Cooking*. She serves as Autism One's consulting chef, is on the advisory board of The University of Chicago Celiac Disease Center and is an Autism Research Institute cooking instructor and consultant.

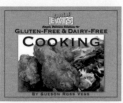

Vess is co-founder of Cumin and Clove, a vegan, gluten-free, allergy-friendly packaged food business that offers simple Indian food for American home cooks.

Special Eats: Simple, Delicious Solutions for Gluten & Dairy Free Cooking is available at LivingWithout.com.

Where to find Sueson Vess:
specialeats.com
cuminandclove.com

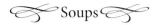

SOUPS

Sueson's
Tomato Vegetable Soup
Serves 8

Eating with the seasons allows you to change this soup depending on readily available vegetables or family preferences. From zucchini to kale or eggplant and fennel, this soup will become your signature dish. Tomatoes and other red foods are rich in the phytonutrients lycopene and anthocyanin that benefit the heart and circulatory system by helping build healthy cells. The more vegetables introduced, the more optimal phytonutrients, so eat the colors of the rainbow.

Ingredients
1 small onion, diced
1 clove garlic, sliced
1 tablespoon olive oil
1 bunch kale, ribs removed and chopped, about 4 cups (may substitute spinach or Swiss chard)
2 medium zucchini, diced
Optional extra vegetables: fennel bulb, thinly sliced; mushrooms, chopped; bell peppers, chopped; eggplant, small dice (about 6 cups total vegetables and greens)
1 (28-32 ounce) can or jar crushed tomatoes in sauce
1 teaspoon dried oregano
½ teaspoon fennel seeds
½ teaspoon salt
¼ teaspoon black pepper
2 cups gluten-free, dairy-free chicken or vegetable broth

Sautéing the Vegetables
Sauté onion and garlic in olive oil in a large skillet over medium heat until soft. Add kale and sauté until wilted and reduced in volume. Add zucchini and any other vegetables and sauté for about 15 minutes.

Fresh, local vegetables pack the most nutrition, and taste the best. Over-ripe or bruised vegetables are fine for soup — and they save you money.

In a rush? Frozen vegetables are another good nutritional source and a great time-saver.

For a spicier soup, add a pinch of red pepper flakes or ½ teaspoon chipotle chili powder.

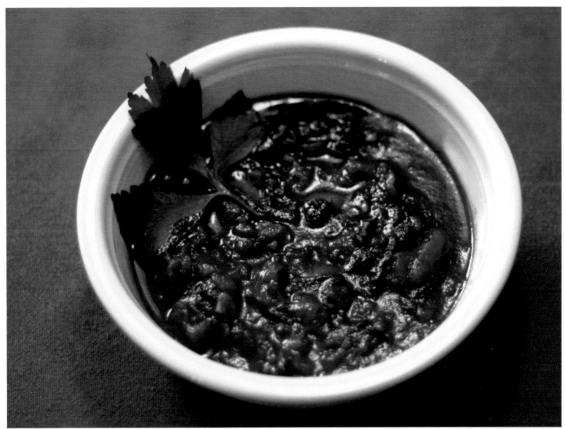
Tomato Vegetable Soup

Finishing Up
Add tomatoes and seasonings to the vegetables and bring to simmer.
Add broth and continue to cook uncovered for at least 15 minutes.
(Longer cooking time thickens soup and enhances flavor.)

To the Table
Taste and adjust seasoning. Serve warm.

Each serving contains 79 calories, 2g total fat, 0g saturated fat, 0g trans fat, 0mg cholesterol, 527mg sodium, 13g carbohydrate, 3g fiber, 1g sugars, 4g protein.

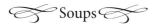
Sueson's
Creamy Mushroom Soup
Serves 8

An autism group asked me to create a healthy Alfredo sauce free of gluten, dairy, soy and corn; if the sauce contained hidden mushrooms, all the better. The sauce was fabulous on gluten-free pasta, over zucchini ribbon "noodles" and more. By adding chicken broth, the sauce became a healthy mushroom soup. Mushrooms contain important B vitamins often missing in the gluten-free diet. Asian mushrooms, like shiitake, maitake and oyster, have more phytonutrients and beta-glucans that help stimulate the immune system. This recipe contains nuts but it can be made nut-free.*

Ingredients
1 tablespoon olive oil
½ cup minced shallots
2 cloves garlic, minced, optional
4 cups chopped mushrooms, shiitake, crimini or a blend
6 tablespoons freshly squeezed lemon juice
¼ teaspoon ground nutmeg
½ teaspoon salt, more to taste
¼ teaspoon freshly ground black pepper
Pinch cayenne pepper, more or less to taste
1 cup raw unsalted almonds,* soaked overnight or at least 8 hours in purified water
1 cup raw unsalted cashew pieces,* soaked in hot water for 30 minutes
½ cup unsalted pine nuts,* soaked in hot water for 30 minutes
4 cups gluten-free, dairy-free chicken, beef or vegetable broth

Sautéing Ingredients
Heat oil in a large saucepan and sauté shallots, garlic and mushrooms over medium heat until beginning to color, about 10 minutes. Add lemon juice and scrape up any brown bits on the bottom of the pan. Add nutmeg, salt, pepper and cayenne. Remove from heat.

Making the Nut "Cream"
Drain almonds, cashews and pine nuts, discarding soaking liquid. Place

A great selection of mushroooms, both fresh and dried, is available in the produce section of most stores.

*For **Nut-Free Mushroom Soup,** omit the almonds, cashews and pine nuts. Add 2½ cups non-dairy yogurt or 2½ cups cooked, drained and puréed white beans, preferably cannellini beans.

Lemon juice or another acidic liquid like vinegar helps loosen all the flavorful bits from the pan, adding delicious richness to the soup.

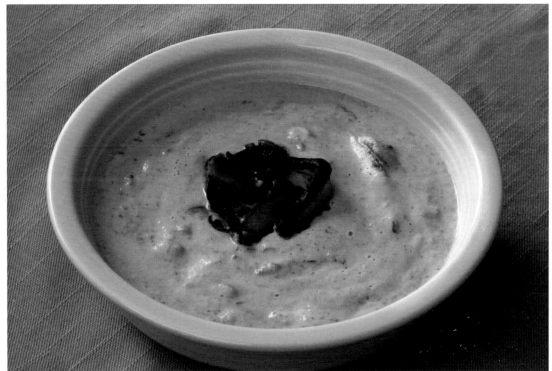

Creamy Mushroom Soup

in a blender in 2 batches, adding ½ to 1 cup fresh water per batch. Do not add too much water as you want the nut "cream" to be fairly thick. Blend until very smooth consistency is reached, about 2 minutes.

Putting It Together
Add mushroom-shallot mixture to nut cream and puree. Leave some of the mushrooms chunky, if desired.

Finishing Up
Return mixture to saucepan and add broth. Bring to simmer. Taste and adjust seasoning. Serve warm.

Store leftover soup for up to 3 days in the refrigerator.

Each serving contains 253 calories, 21g total fat, 2g saturated fat, 0g trans fat, 0mg cholesterol, 613mg sodium, 13g carbohydrate, 3g fiber, 3g sugars, 8g protein.

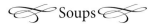

Sueson's
Kale and White Bean Soup
Serves 8

Kale, my favorite super-green food, has unmatched beneficial qualities, ranging from its many antioxidants and flavonoids to its anti-inflammatory and detoxifying abilities. When combined with cannellini beans, kale creates a hearty and comforting soup that is as good for you as it is tasty. Don't tell your kids!

Ingredients
2 tablespoons olive oil
1 small red onion, finely chopped
3 cloves garlic, minced
4 stalks celery, thinly sliced
2 bunches kale, ribs removed, chopped, about 8 cups
3 plum tomatoes, chopped
6 cups gluten-free, dairy-free vegetable or chicken broth
2 (15-ounce) cans cannellini beans, rinsed and drained
1 bay leaf
1 teaspoon dried thyme
½ teaspoon sea salt
½ teaspoon pepper

Sautéing the Vegetables
In large stockpot, heat olive oil over medium-high heat. Add onion, garlic and celery and sauté until softened, about 5 to 7 minutes, stirring occasionally. Add kale and sauté for 2 minutes until kale has wilted and is reduced to a quarter of its original volume.

Adding the Broth and Finishing Up
Add tomatoes and stir until coated with oil. Stir in broth, beans, bay leaf, thyme, salt and pepper.

Simmer for 20 minutes, covered. Remove bay leaf before serving. Taste and adjust seasoning.

Each serving contains 232 calories, 5g total fat, 1g saturated fat, 0g trans fat, 0mg cholesterol, 904mg sodium, 37g carbohydrate, 9g fiber, 2g sugars, 14g protein.

Cannellini beans from a can have the same nutritional benefits as dried beans but without the work. Always rinse and drain canned beans before using. Add to salads and soups for a nutritional boost.

No time to make your own vegetable or chicken broth? Some packaged varieties are gluten-free and dairy-free. See Shopping List (page 189).

Pile on the kale. It reduces to about a quarter of its original volume when cooked.

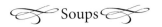

Sueson's
Thai Coconut Soup
Serves 6

Coconut milk, lemongrass and ginger are an amazing flavor combination, turning a novice cook into an exotic Thai chef. This soup can be enjoyed by vegetarians and chicken or fish lovers and is also a great sauce to poach fish or to serve over grilled chicken or fish. The interesting combination of spicy, sour and sweet flavors melds into the creamy coconut, creating an exotic vacation in a bowl.

Ingredients
2 (13.5-ounce) cans unsweetened coconut milk
2 stalks fresh lemongrass, cut into 3-inch pieces or
1 package fresh lemongrass or
3 pieces dried lemongrass (no cutting)
¼ cup minced shallots
1 (2-inch) piece fresh ginger root, peeled and minced
1 lime, zest and juice
2 cups gluten-free, dairy-free vegetable or chicken broth
2 cups combination chopped zucchini, bell peppers and carrots
OR 2 cups bite-size pieces cooked chicken and
1½ cups sliced bok choy
OR 1½ cups (2-inch pieces) salmon (or other firm fish) and 2 cups
fresh spinach or Swiss chard, chopped
½ teaspoon salt
¼ teaspoon chili pepper flakes
½ cup fresh cilantro, chopped, for garnish
1 lime, cut into 8 wedges, for garnish

Preparing the Broth
Combine coconut milk, lemongrass, shallots, ginger, lime zest and juice in large saucepan over medium heat and bring to a simmer. Reduce heat to low and let simmer uncovered for 25 minutes. Add broth and return to simmer. Remove lemongrass and discard.

Preparing the Vegetables
Add vegetables, chicken or fish to the saucepan. Cooking time varies. For vegetables, simmer 10 to 15 minutes or until carrots are tender. For

Fresh lemongrass stalks are available in the produce section of many grocery stores. Look for it where other packaged fresh herbs are sold.

If using fresh lemongrass stalks, slice off the root end and cut the stalks into 3-inch pieces. Tie pieces together with kitchen twine for easier removal after cooking.

Dried lemongrass is available from Thai Kitchen. Look for it in the ethnnic food section of your supermarket.

If using dried lemongrass, use two to three 3-inch pieces. Remove with a slotted spoon before serving.

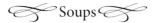

chicken, add chicken and bok choy and simmer for 5 to 7 minutes. For fish, add raw salmon and simmer for 6 minutes. Add spinach or Swiss chard and simmer an additional 2 minutes. Add salt and chili pepper flakes. Taste and adjust seasoning.

Finishing Up
Ladle into bowls and top with fresh cilantro. Serve with a wedge of lime.

Each serving contains 343 calories, 32g total fat, 27g saturated fat, 0g trans fat, 0mg cholesterol, 562mg sodium, 13g carbohydrate, 2g fiber, 4g sugars, 3g protein.

HOMEMADE BROTH
Why bother making homemade broth when there are commercial gluten-free, dairy-free options available?

The Answer Is Simple
Homemade means better flavor, increased nutrition and control over your ingredients, including the amount of added sodium. You won't find MSG or mystery items like hydrolyzed yeast or unnamed spices in homemade broth unless you choose to add them.

Waste Not and Save Money
Once you get into the routine of making your own broth, you can save money by using produce and meat you might ordinarily throw away—thick broccoli stalks, green tops of leeks, mushroom stems, a leftover turkey or chicken carcass or beef bones from dinner. For quick and easy broth, make it in your crockpot overnight. To store unused broth, refrigerate it in a covered container for up to 3 days or freeze it in portion-size containers or ice cube trays for up to 3 months.

The recipes for **Sueson's Homemade Broths** are on pages 86 and 87.

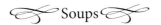

Sueson's
Chicken Tortilla Soup
Serves 6

For a list of companies ofering gluten-free, non-dairy cheese alternatives, see Shopping List, page 189.

Mexican food was a favorite in my BC (before celiac) days. Now AD (after diagnosis), I still enjoy Mexican food but need good detective skills to assure that it is free of gluten, dairy and other offending ingredients. So it's back to the kitchen where I know my food is both safe and delicious. This soup couldn't be easier and gets rave reviews from young and old. My granddaughter says it's because it contains a secret ingredient—chocolate!

Ingredients
1 cup prepared gluten-free salsa
1 (28-32 ounce) can or jar crushed tomatoes in sauce
2 cups gluten-free, dairy-free chicken broth
2 teaspoons chili powder blend or single chili powder, like ground ancho chili
1 tablespoon unsweetened cocoa powder
½ teaspoon ground cinnamon
2½ cups bite-size pieces cooked chicken or turkey
3 gluten-free soft corn tortillas, cut into 1-inch squares (to slightly thicken soup)
½ teaspoon salt
¼ teaspoon freshly ground black pepper

Garnishes
1 ripe avocado, peeled and cubed
Gluten-free tortilla chips
Chopped cilantro
Gluten-free hot sauce
Non-dairy Pepper Jack-style shreds, optional

Combining the Ingredients
Combine salsa, tomatoes, broth, chili powder, cocoa, cinnamon, chicken and tortillas in a large stockpot over medium heat. Bring to simmer and let cook for 15 minutes.

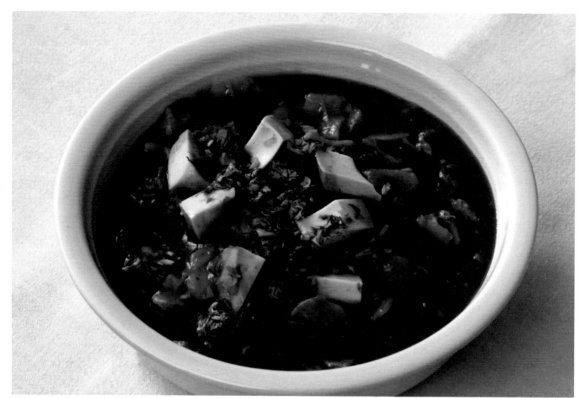

Chicken Tortilla Soup

Finishing Up

Add salt and pepper and taste; adjust seasonings. Serve warm, topped with avocado, tortilla chips and cilantro. Serve hot sauce and cheese on the side.

Each serving contains 240 calories, 8g total fat, 2g saturated fat, 0g trans fat, 50mg cholesterol, 1029mg sodium, 22g carbohydrate, 6g fiber, 2g sugars, 24g protein.

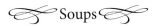 Soups

Sueson's
Sweet Potato Chowder
Serves 8

For variation, add 1 apple, thinly sliced or 2 cups peeled and cubed butternut squash to roasting vegetables.

As a child, I didn't care for sweet potatoes. Now, I can't get enough of this amazing powerhouse of flavor and nutrient-dense goodness. Sweet potatoes can replace white potatoes in everything from French fries to mashed potatoes, potato salads and, of course, soup.

Chowder, which is typically a thick, cream-based soup, is a perfect foundation for a gluten-free, dairy-free translation and is packed with health-giving nutrients. Beta carotene, which our bodies convert into vitamin A, gives sweet potatoes their orange color. Vitamin A builds a strong immune system but this fat-soluble nutrient needs fat to realize these benefits. So remember to include a little fat with your vitamin A-rich veggies.

Ingredients
1 large onion, coarsely chopped
2 carrots, coarsely chopped
4 large sweet potatoes, peeled and cut into 1-inch pieces
2-3 tablespoons olive oil
1 teaspoon ground ginger
½ teaspoon ground turmeric
½ teaspoon ground nutmeg
½ teaspoon ground cinnamon
¼ teaspoon white pepper
4 cups gluten-free, dairy-free vegetable or chicken broth
2 cups non-dairy unflavored milk of choice
½ teaspoon salt

Garnish
1 large apple, cored and thinly sliced (toss in 2 teaspoons lemon or lime juice to keep from turning brown)
¼ cup ground pepita seeds (shelled pumpkin seeds)
Gluten-free bacon crumbles, optional

Getting Started
Preheat oven to 400°F.

Roasting the Vegetables
In a large, heavy roasting pan, toss onion, carrots and sweet potatoes

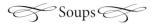
in olive oil and roast in preheated oven for 20 minutes, stirring halfway through cooking.

Preparing the Broth

Place roasted vegetables in a large stockpot. Add ginger, turmeric, nutmeg, cinnamon, white pepper and broth and simmer for 15 minutes or until the vegetables are very soft. Stir in non-dairy milk and salt and heat to low boil.

Puréeing the Soup

In a blender or food processor, puree the soup in batches. Do not fill blender more than half full and cover container with a dish towel before turning the machine on to avoid being burned by splattering liquid.

Finishing Up

Taste and adjust seasoning. Serve warm. Garnish with apple slices and sprinkle with ground pepita seeds and bacon crumbles, if used.

Get better flavor, increased nutrition and control over your ingredients, (especially the amount of added sodium) by making your own broth. See Chicken, Turkey, Beef Broth, page 86, and Vegetable Broth, page 87.

Each serving contains 188 calories, 8g total fat, 1g saturated fat, 0g trans fat, 0mg cholesterol, 680mg sodium, 27g carbohydrate, 4g fiber, 10g sugars, 5g protein.

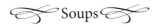

Sueson's
Cantaloupe Gazpacho
Serves 6 to 8

Gazpacho, a Spanish-inspired cold soup, typically includes bread or nuts for thickness and is often tomato-based. This gluten, dairy and tomato-free version uses cantaloupe, creating a slightly sweet, fruity rendition of a traditional favorite. This cold soup is refreshing in the summer but it provides cooling relief to a spicy entrée any time of the year.

Ingredients
1 cantaloupe, peeled, seeded and cut into chunks
¼ cup fresh lemon or lime juice
½ cup Cashew Cream,* or ⅓ cup sunflower seed butter blended with ½ cup water
1 cup gluten-free, dairy-free vegetable or chicken broth or water
¼ teaspoon ground nutmeg
Pinch of salt

Combining the Ingredients
Add cantaloupe, lemon or lime juice, Cashew Cream, broth, nutmeg and salt to a blender or food processor and puree until smooth.

Chilling and Serving
Chill until ready to enjoy.

*If nuts are tolerated, Cashew Cream is a good non-dairy replacement for cream or sour cream in both sweet and savory dishes.

To make 1 cup Cashew Cream, cover ⅔ cup raw, unsalted cashews with boiling water and let sit 5 minutes. Puree mixture in a blender until it is the consistency of cream. Add more water, if needed, to produce a smooth consistency.

If using sunflower seed butter, you may choose to add sweetener of choice, to taste.

Each serving contains 139calories, 7g total fat, 1g saturated fat, 0g trans fat, 0mg cholesterol, 246mg sodium, 16g carbohydrate, 3g fiber, 4g protein.

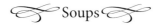
Apple Fennel Soup
Serves 4
(RECIPE BY SUESON VESS)

The health benefits of chicken broth enhance this creamy non-dairy soup. It's full of anti-oxidants and vitamin C, as well as flavonoids like quercetin found in many natural cold remedies. Serve hot, garnished with chopped chives or red apple cut into matchsticks. (Toss apple pieces with fresh lemon juice to prevent browning.)

Ingredients
2 medium fennel bulbs, stalk and fronds removed, chopped (about 5 cups)
1 large onion, chopped
2 tablespoons extra-virgin olive oil
¼ cup Madeira wine, Port, apple cider or apple juice
2 cups gluten-free, dairy-free chicken broth
2 large apples (Granny Smith or other firm, tart apple), peeled, cored and diced
1 bay leaf
1 teaspoon dried thyme
¼ teaspoon ground nutmeg
½ teaspoon salt and pepper, to taste

Sautéing
In a large, heavy-bottom stockpot, sauté fennel and onion in olive oil until softened and slightly browned, about 15 minutes.

Flavoring the Broth
Add wine and let cook for a minute. Add chicken broth, apples, bay leaf and thyme. Simmer uncovered for 20 minutes or until apples and fennel are soft.

Finishing Up
Remove bay leaf and carefully puree soup in small batches in a blender or food processor.

For velvety-smooth texture, pass soup through a food mill or strain.

Stir in nutmeg and add salt and pepper, to taste.

Each serving contains 221 calories, 9g total fat, 1g saturated fat, 0g trans fat, 4mg cholesterol, 34g carbohydrate, 526mg sodium, 6g fiber, 5g protein.

For vegetarian soup, replace chicken broth with gluten-free, dairy-free vegetable broth.

Chicken, Turkey or Beef Broth
Makes 3 quarts
(RECIPE BY SUESON VESS)

Mineral-rich chicken, turkey or beef broth is the base for many soups, sauces and gravies. Aside from the wonderful taste, this nutrition-packed liquid is beneficial for steaming vegetables, cooking gluten-free grains, like rice and quinoa, or for use whenever a savory liquid is recommended. Add ½ cup broth to 2 cups tomato-based red sauces to boost flavor and nutrition. Broth can be made from raw or cooked bones, although there are more minerals available from raw bones.

Ingredients
3-3½ pounds chicken or turkey pieces, mostly backs and wings
(do not use chicken/turkey liver) or
6 pounds beef bones,
about half with meat left on bones
2 yellow or white onions, quartered
1 leek, including green part, cut in quarters
6 carrots (unpeeled), cut in large chunks
6 celery stalks, cut in large chunks
Additional vegetables, such as sweet potatoes, broccoli or others, to taste

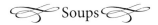

12 cups cold water
2 bay leaves
Handful of parsley stems and/or
fresh thyme sprigs
½ teaspoon whole black peppercorns
1 kombu* "stick"
2 tablespoons cider vinegar or fresh lemon
juice for chicken or turkey broth
or ¼ cup for beef broth
Salt, to taste
3-4 dried juniper berries, optional

Combining the Ingredients
Place chicken, turkey, or beef in a large stock-pot over medium heat. Add vegetables. Add enough cold water to cover bones, at least 12 cups. Add bay leaves, parsley or thyme, pep-percorns, kombu, vinegar, salt and juniper and slowly bring to a boil.

Simmering
Reduce heat to low and gently simmer for 3 to 4 hours (5 to 6 hours for beef broth). As the broth cooks, skim any impurities that rise to the surface.

Finishing Up
Remove chicken, turkey or beef pieces and dis-card. Strain the broth through a fine sieve into another container and discard vegetable sol-ids. Skim off excess fat. If not using the broth immediately, place the container in a sink full of ice water and stir to cool. When cool, cover and refrigerate or freeze.

> *Kombu, a type of seaweed, is available in the Asian food section of most grocery stores.

Vegetable Broth
Makes 2 quarts
(RECIPE BY SUESON VESS)

Homemade means better flavor, increased nutrition and control over your ingredients.

Ingredients
10 cups water
2 potatoes, red, white or sweet, unpeeled
and quartered
2 onions, quartered
8 mushrooms
2 leeks, including green part, cut in quarters
2 carrots, cut into 2-inch pieces
2 celery ribs, cut into 2-inch pieces
2 cloves garlic or 1 small shallot, roughly cut
½ bunch fresh flat-leaf parsley stems
(reserve leaves for other use)
1 kombu* "stick"
8 whole peppercorns
4 whole cloves
1 bay leaf
1 teaspoon sea salt

Combining the Ingredients
Place all ingredients, except salt, in a large stockpot and bring to a boil. Reduce heat and simmer uncovered for at least 1½ to 2 hours. Longer cooking time makes for richer flavor and nutrition.

Finishing Up
Remove broth from heat and strain it through a fine sieve into another container, discarding solids. Taste broth and add salt, to taste.

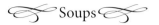

Lamb Porcupines in Broth
Serves 4 to 6
(RECIPE BY SUESON VESS)

Delicious lamb meatballs are transformed into floating porcupine balls when cooked in simmering broth. This hearty soup is high in protein and minerals, especially vitamin B12 and zinc, important for immune function. Spinach adds vitamins A, C and K and is a good source of folic acid, magnesium and iron.

Ingredients
1 pound ground lamb, preferably organic, grass-fed
1 (3-inch) piece fresh ginger root, peeled and finely minced
2 garlic cloves or 1 small shallot, finely minced
3 tablespoons fresh cilantro, chopped
½ teaspoon ground turmeric
¼ teaspoon ground fennel seed
½ teaspoon sea salt
¼ teaspoon freshly ground black pepper
¼ cup raw basmati rice
6 cups gluten-free, dairy-free chicken or beef broth
2 cups fresh spinach, coarsely chopped (leave whole if baby spinach)
½ teaspoon sea salt

Combining the Ingredients
In a large bowl, combine lamb, ginger, garlic, cilantro, turmeric, fennel seed, ½ teaspoon salt, pepper and rice. Do not over-mix. Form into walnut-size meatballs and set aside.

Finishing Up
Bring broth to a rolling boil in a large (6 quarts or larger) pot. Add meatballs and simmer covered for 15 minutes. Add spinach and ½ teaspoon salt and cook for an additional 2 minutes. Taste and adjust seasoning.

Each serving contains 260 calories, 18g total fat, 8g saturated fat, 0g trans fat, 55mg cholesterol, 601mg sodium, 8g carbohydrate, 1g fiber, 16g protein.

Roasted Beet Soup
Serves 6 to 8
(RECIPE BY SUESON VESS)

Beets are a good source of folate, potassium and iron. They derive their rich jewel-tone color in part from cancer-fighting betacyanin. High in natural sugar and low in calories, beets are particularly delicious when roasted. Serve this soup hot, topped with a dollop of non-dairy plain yogurt.

Ingredients
3 pounds fresh red beets, trimmed, peeled and cut into pieces
1 large onion, chopped
2 carrots, chopped
1 red or yellow bell pepper, chopped
2 tablespoons extra-virgin olive oil
2 cups apple cider
2 cups gluten-free, dairy-free chicken or vegetable broth
1 teaspoon dried tarragon
½ teaspoon each, salt and pepper, to taste

Getting Started
Preheat oven to 400°F.

Roasting the Vegetables
Toss beets, onion, carrots and bell pepper in olive oil and spread in a single layer in a large roasting pan. Cook in preheated oven for 45 minutes or until beets and other vegetables are softened.

Making the Soup
Add apple cider, chicken broth and roasted

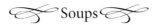
vegetables to a large stockpot and simmer for 15 minutes. Add tarragon and salt and pepper, to taste.

Finishing Up
Carefully puree soup in small batches in a blender or food processor. Add water or additional broth to thin to desired consistency. Serve hot.

Each serving contains 170 calories, 4g total fat, 1g saturated fat, 0g trans fat, 2mg cholesterol, 29g carbohydrate, 303mg sodium, 6g fiber, 5g protein.

Pumpkin Soup with Apple Croutons
Serves 8
(RECIPE BY BETH HILLSON)

Here's a delightful way to start a special meal. Serve this soup as an elegant first course that will wow your guests at the holidays or any time of year. Ladle into pretty bowls or hollowed-out, cooked mini-pumpkins. Garnish with Apple Croutons and a dollop of non-dairy yogurt.

Ingredients
2 tablespoons olive oil
1 large leek, trimmed, chopped and rinsed thoroughly
1 tablespoon minced fresh garlic
2 tablespoons minced fresh ginger root
2 teaspoons ground cinnamon
2 (15-ounce) cans pure pumpkin puree
1 teaspoon salt
¼ teaspoon freshly ground black pepper
2 cups gluten-free, dairy-free chicken broth
2 cups apple juice
½ cup unflavored yogurt or non-dairy alternative, more for garnish
Apple Croutons, for garnish

Sautéing and Cooking the Vegetables
Place olive oil in a large saucepan and warm over medium heat. Sauté the leek until soft and cooked down. Add the garlic and ginger and sauté 1 minute. Add the cinnamon and sauté briefly, about 30 seconds, or just until it gives off its fragrance. Add pumpkin, salt, pepper, chicken broth and apple juice. Bring to a boil. Reduce to a simmer and cook the soup for 15 minutes, covered.

Making It Creamy
Remove soup from heat and process with an immersion blender (or in batches in a blender) until smooth. Season with additional salt and pepper, to taste. Stir in ½ cup yogurt until combined.

Finishing Up
Divide soup evenly among 8 bowls. Garnish each with 2 Apple Croutons and a dollop of yogurt. Serve warm.

Each serving of soup contains 125 calories, 5g total fat, 1g saturated fat, 0g trans fat, mg cholesterol, 320mg sodium, 20g carbohydrate, 4g fiber, 3g protein.

Apple Croutons
Makes 16 slices
These can be prepared ahead and refrigerated for several days. If time is short, use a commercial brand of apple chips.

Ingredients
2 apples, such as Granny Smith or McIntosh, cored
⅓ cup firmly packed light brown sugar

Getting Started
Preheat oven to 300°F. Line a baking sheet with parchment paper.

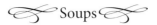

Preparing the Apples
Cut apples into 8 slices. Spread slices in one layer on prepared baking sheet and sprinkle evenly with brown sugar.

Baking the Apples
Place on middle rack of preheated oven and bake 20 minutes or until golden. Transfer immediately to a rack to cool.

Each crouton contains 30 calories, 0g total fat, 0g saturated fat, 0g trans fat, 0mg cholesterol, 0mg sodium, 8g carbohydrate, 0g fiber, 0g protein.

Turkey & White Tea Noodle Soup
Serves 4
(RECIPE BY MATTHEW KADEY)

Why just drink tea when you can cook with it? Tea leaves, which are teeming with disease-fighting antioxidants, can be sprinkled into rubs, soups, stews and even desserts for wonderful flavor and an added health boost. The delicate nature of white tea broth allows the robust flavor of kale, lemongrass and sesame oil to shine in this gluten-free, dairy-free soup.

Ingredients
2 (6-ounce) uncooked boneless turkey breasts, cut into strips
2 tablespoons olive oil
4 ounces gluten-free Asian rice noodles
6 cups water
3 teaspoons loose-leaf white tea (or 2 white tea bags)
1 (1-inch) piece ginger, peeled and thinly sliced
1 stalk lemongrass, outside leaves removed and finely chopped
1 cup frozen peas or shelled edamame, frozen, optional
1 cup mushrooms, thinly sliced
2 cups kale, chopped
½ teaspoon sea salt
1 teaspoon sesame oil
Freshly ground black pepper, for garnish
Fresh cilantro, for garnish

Preparing the Turkey
Cook turkey and oil over medium heat in a skillet until no longer pink. Remove from heat and let stand.

Making the Noodles
Prepare noodles according to package directions. Drain and set aside.

Making the Tea
In a large pot, combine 6 cups water with white tea and ginger. Heat until water is just about to reach a boil. Remove from heat and let steep for about 5 minutes.

Strain liquid tea to remove leaves. Return ginger pieces to liquid. Add lemongrass and heat until mixture returns to a boil.

Putting It Together
Drop frozen peas into pot and cover. Reduce heat and simmer for 3 minutes.

Add mushrooms, kale and salt and cook an additional 2 minutes. Add rice noodles, turkey pieces and sesame oil. Stir well.

Finishing Up
Place soup in serving bowls. Top with ground pepper and cilantro. Serve hot.

Each serving contains 307 calories, 6g total fat, 1g saturated fat, 0g trans fat, 36mg cholesterol, 39g carbohydrate, 1220mg sodium, 4g fiber, 25g protein.

MAIN COURSE

"No need to ask, 'What's for dinner?'
From simple to elegant, this chapter of kid- and family-favorite
recipes has you covered."

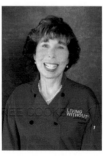

Recipes by
Beth Hillson
and other celebrity chefs

Beth Hillson

Glastonbury, Connecticut

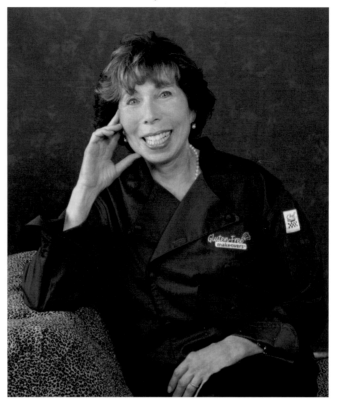

"I am the champion of substitution! The glass is not empty if you arm yourself
with friendly substitutions and serve the same delicious, safe version to everyone."

When I was diagnosed with celiac disease 35 years ago, I went to culinary school to better understand how food was prepared. I discovered I could remake the recipes as long as I maintained the ratio of ingredients in the original recipe. I replaced regular flour with gluten-free flour and the results were always delicious. As food editor at *Living Without* magazine, I am always thinking "substitution" when making a recipe and these basic principles, discovered 35 years ago, still hold true. We regularly replace the gluten and dairy (and often the eggs) in our recipes with yummy results.

These days, I think of myself as the champion of substitution. But truthfully, it's about knowing the ingredients to replace. For that I keep

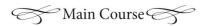

a running list of suitable alternatives. I know, for instance, that some butter alternatives contain casein while others are vegan and completely dairy-free. I know that these dairy-free butter substitutions can be cut and frozen before adding to a recipe to make flakier pie crust and cookies. And I can list the alternatives for milk in order of the ones with the highest protein—soy, hemp, almond, rice and potato—for starters.

When readers write to *Living Without* with a lengthy list of ingredients they must avoid, I suggest they make a list of the ingredients they *can* have, and keep those in mind every time they want to make a recipe. It's empowering. It makes them feel like the world is full of possibilities. After all, the glass is not empty if you arm yourself with friendly alternatives.

Substitution is my mantra. When I see a yummy-looking dessert, a loaf of bread, a stack of pancakes or when I read a recipe that sounds delicious, I immediately go to my stockpile of replacements to make the dish safe for my diet. As a result, I never feel like I go without. I always have an abundance of great foods to eat.

And I don't hesitate to serve what I've made to all my guests without mentioning that the food is gluten and dairy-free. Gluten-free food has become so tasty, there's no need to make two varieties. The sophisticated flour blends that we make today with finely ground rice flour and nutrient-dense flours like amaranth and sorghum make it possible to create fabulous dishes without gluten. We are fortunate, indeed, to have so many choices.

Beth Hillson is the founder of Gluten-Free Pantry, one of the first gluten-free companies in the United States.

A food writer and cooking instructor, Hillson is food editor of *Living Without* and author of *Gluten-Free Makeovers* (Da Capo Press).

Where to find Beth Hillson:
glutenfreemakeovers.com
LivingWithout.com

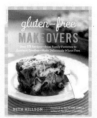

Gluten-Free Makeovers is available at LivingWithout.com

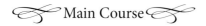

MAIN COURSE

Beth's
El Diablo Chicken
Serves 4

This is adapted from a wonderful dish I enjoyed at Evil Dave's Grill in Jasper, Alberta. Don't be concerned by its name. This dish is more flavorful than spicy.

Ingredients
4 large boneless, skinless chicken breasts
(about 1–1½ pounds)

Marinade
¼ cup olive oil
1 tablespoon chili powder
1 tablespoon minced garlic
Juice of 1 large lime

Main Dish
1 tablespoon olive oil
1 medium yellow onion, diced
2 vine-ripened tomatoes, diced, or 1 (15-ounce) can diced
tomatoes, drained
½-1 teaspoon chipotle chili powder, to taste
2 cups gluten-free, dairy-free chicken broth
¼-½ cup heavy cream or coconut milk, optional
½ cup frozen corn kernels, thawed
½ cup canned black beans, rinsed and drained
1½ cups cooked Jasmine rice

Garnish
1-2 ripe avocados, thinly sliced
2 scallions, top third removed, coarsely chopped

Getting Started
Combine marinade ingredients and add chicken breasts. Stir to coat and let stand, refrigerated, for at least 3 hours.

Chipotle chili powder adds great flavor to this dish and some heat, too. Use a little or a lot, depending on your preference.

Pick avocados that are firm but yield to gentle pressure. If they're mushy to touch, they're too ripe to slice.

Hard avocados will ripen on the counter after a couple of days if time permits.

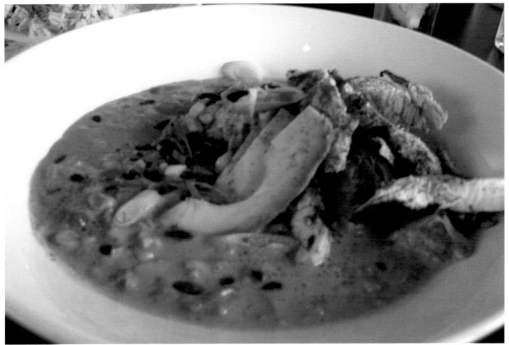

El Diablo Chicken

Sautéing the Vegetables and Reducing the Broth
Heat 1 tablespoon olive oil in a medium saucepan. Sauté the onion and tomatoes for 2 to 3 minutes or until onion is translucent. Add chipotle powder and sauté briefly. Then add the chicken broth and simmer until reduced by half.

Grill the chicken while the broth is reducing.

Grilling the Chicken
While the mixture is simmering, preheat a grill to medium high and grill the chicken on both sides until centers are no longer pink.* Remove from heat. Let cool slightly and slice each fillet diagonally to yield 5 to 6 slices each.

*If a grill is not available, broil chicken breasts in the oven.

Finishing Up and Serving
Add the cream to the reduced chicken broth mixture and simmer 2 to 3 minutes. Remove from heat.

Fold in corn and black beans.

Divide rice among 4 plates. Spoon a portion of the tomato mixture over the rice. Fan out chicken slices over the top and garnish with avocado slices and a sprinkle of chopped scallions.

Can't have dairy? Replace cream with coconut milk.

Each serving contains 563 calories, 30g total fat, 6g saturated fat, 0g trans fat, 75mg cholesterol, 600mg sodium, 43g carbohydrate, 8g fiber, 7g sugars, 34g protein.

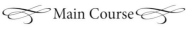

Beth's
Meatball Hero Sandwiches
Serves 8

Makes 2 to 3 dozen meatballs. Roasted meatballs may be frozen.

Not so many years ago, this family favorite would have been off limits to those on a gluten-free diet as bread crumbs and good gluten-free rolls were not readily available. Thanks to the availability of both, this popular dish is now an easy choice. The meatballs are also great with spaghetti or other gluten-free pasta. These meatballs can be made egg-free.*

Ingredients
2 tablespoons olive oil
1 large onion, chopped
3 cloves garlic, minced
1 teaspoon salt
2 pounds lean ground beef
2 hot gluten-free sausages, crumbled
¾ cup gluten-free bread crumbs
3 large eggs,* lightly beaten
¼ cup water
Salt and pepper, to taste
4 cups gluten-free marinara sauce
8 gluten-free hoagie, hot dog or hamburger rolls
Grated cheese or non-dairy cheese, optional

*For **Egg-Free Meatballs,** omit 3 eggs. Combine 3 tablespoons flax meal with 9 tablespoons warm water; let sit 5 minutes until slightly thickened. Then add to recipe to replace 3 eggs.

Getting Started
Preheat oven to 425°F.

Sautéing the Onions
Heat olive oil in a medium skillet over medium heat. Add onions. Sauté until softened and lightly brown, about 5 minutes. Add garlic and sauté 1 minute. Add salt. Set aside.

Making the Meatballs
Mix together ground beef, sausage, bread crumbs, eggs, water, salt and pepper until thoroughly combined. Fold in onion mixture. Roll into golf ball-size balls and set in a roasting pan in a single layer.

Baking the Meatballs
Place in preheated oven and bake 15 minutes. Drain off excess fat and juices. Turn meatballs and roast another 15 minutes.

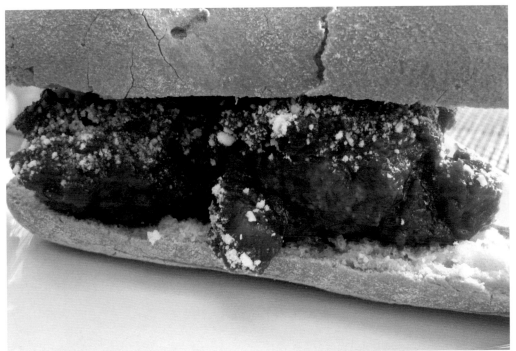

Meatball Hero Sandwich

Finishing Up

Heat marinara sauce in a large saucepan. Add meatballs and simmer briefly.

Toast the rolls. Cut in half and spoon meatballs and sauce over the rolls. Top with grated cheese, if desired.

Make your own bread crumbs by grinding the ends of gluten-free loaves in a food processor.

Each serving contains 421 calories, 35g total fat, 13g saturated fat, 2g trans fat, 140mg cholesterol, 131mg sodium, 7g carbohydrate, 0g fiber, 1g sugars, 18g protein.

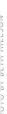

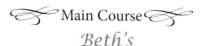

Beth's
Marinated Beef Kebabs
Serves 6

These are great for a summer party. The trick is to cut the beef in small cubes so people don't need knives. Keep an eye on them so they don't overcook.

Ingredients
1½ pounds beef sirloin, cut into 1-inch cubes
Olive oil for brushing grill

Marinade
2 tablespoons olive oil
2 teaspoons red wine vinegar
2 teaspoons sweet paprika
1 teaspoon brown sugar
¼ teaspoon red pepper flakes, optional
¼ teaspoon ground cumin
2 cloves garlic, crushed

Kebabs pair nicely with any number of gluten-free condiments and sauces. Use whatever is at hand.

Making the Marinade
Mix marinade ingredients in a large bowl. Add beef cubes. Toss to coat.

Cover and refrigerate at least 2 hours, preferably overnight.

Assembling and Grilling the Kebabs
Soak 12 to 18 bamboo skewers in water for 1 to 2 hours.

For best flavor, marinate the kebabs overnight.

Heat the grill to high. Thread 4 pieces of meat onto each skewer. Brush the grids of the grill with olive oil to prevent the meat from sticking. Grill kebabs about 4 minutes. Turn and grill an additional 2 to 3 minutes, depending on how well done you like your beef. Keep an eye on the kebabs so they do not overcook.

Serving the Kebabs
Arrange kebabs on a platter. Serve hot with Chimichurri Sauce, page 130.

Each serving contains 450 calories, 38g total fat, 6g saturated fat, 0g trans fat, 41mg cholesterol, 653mg sodium, 7g carbohydrate, 1g fiber, 1g sugars, 25g protein.

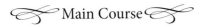

Beth's
Turkey Marsala
Serves 4

This quick dish dresses up leftovers and might even fool family members into thinking you spent a lot of time in the kitchen. Serve with rice or gluten-free noodles. This recipe can be made egg-free.*

Flat gluten-free noodles, labeled tagliatelle or fettucine, are perfect to serve with this dish.

Ingredients
6 slices cooked turkey breast or chicken breast
1 large egg,* lightly beaten, or ¼ cup milk of choice
½ cup cornstarch
2 tablespoons butter or olive oil
2 tablespoons olive oil, divided
Salt and pepper, to taste
2 shallots, finely chopped
½ pound mushrooms, sliced
½ cup gluten-free, dairy-free chicken broth
¼ cup Marsala wine
Shredded mozzarella cheese or non-dairy cheese alternative, optional

Getting Started
Preheat oven to 350°F.

Preparing the Turkey
Dip turkey slices in egg (or milk of choice) and then cornstarch.

In a large skillet, sauté meat in 2 tablespoons butter and 1 tablespoon oil until just browned. Sprinkle with salt and pepper. Arrange meat in a single layer in large glass baking dish.

Finishing Up
Add remaining 1 tablespoon oil to skillet and sauté shallots and mushrooms. Mix in broth and wine and pour mixture over turkey slices. Sprinkle cheese over turkey, if desired.

Place dish uncovered in preheated oven and bake for 20 minutes or until cheese melts. Serve hot over rice or gluten-free noodles.

Each serving contains 223 calories, 5g total fat, 3g saturated fat, 0g trans fat, 15mg cholesterol, 65mg sodium, 12g carbohydrate, 0g fiber, 28g protein.

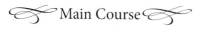 Main Course

Beth's
Chicken and Dumplings

Serves 4

I recently asked people what they missed most after they became gluten-free. The number one answer was Chicken and Dumplings, a comfort food we all equate with nourishing goodness.

Scoop the dumpling dough onto simmering (not boiling) liquid and cover the pot tightly. Don't peek while the dumplings cook. These are best eaten right away but they also make tasty leftovers. These dumplings can be made egg-free.*

Ingredients
4 cups gluten-free, dairy-free chicken broth, more as needed
¼ cup dry sherry or vermouth, optional
1 clove garlic, crushed
1 pound boneless, skinless chicken breasts
Salt and freshly ground pepper
1 medium onion, chopped
2 celery stalks, trimmed and chopped
3 medium carrots, peeled and chopped
3 medium parsnips, peeled and chopped
2 medium potatoes, peeled and cubed
1 teaspoon dried thyme
¾ cup frozen peas, thawed
¼ cup minced fresh parsley leaves

Dumplings
Makes about 12
2 cups *Living Without's* All-Purpose Flour Blend (page xiv)
3 teaspoons baking powder
1 teaspoon xanthan gum
¾ teaspoon salt
2-3 tablespoons minced fresh chives or other fresh herbs
2 tablespoons butter or non-dairy alternative, melted
¾ cup + 2 tablespoons milk of choice
1 large egg,* beaten

Getting Started
Heat the chicken broth to a gentle simmer in a medium saucepan. Add sherry, if used, and garlic.

For quicker preparation, use a gluten-free cooked rotisserie chicken in this recipe.

*For **Egg-Free Dumplings,** omit 1 egg. Combine 1 tablespoon flax meal with 2 tablespoons warm water; let sit for 5 minutes until thickened. Add to recipe to replace 1 egg. If needed, add more water to the dumpling batter, 1 teaspoon at a time, until desired consistency is reached.

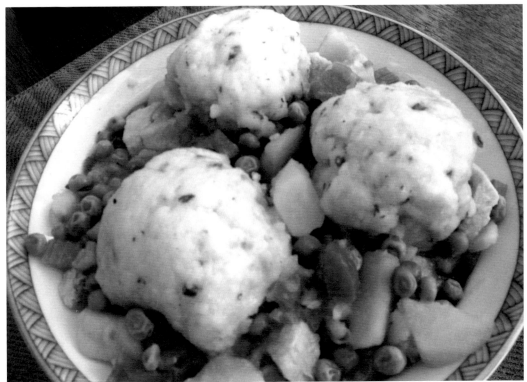

Chicken and Dumplings

Cooking the Chicken
Add chicken breasts and salt and pepper, to taste. Poach covered for 5 minutes.

Using a slotted spoon, remove the breasts and cool. Skim foam off the surface of the liquid. (If using pre-cooked rotisserie chicken, it is not neccessary to cook the chicken.)

Finishing the Broth
Return the pot of chicken broth to medium-high heat.

Add the onion, celery, carrots, parsnips, potatoes, and thyme. Cover and simmer vegetables until just fork tender, about 10 minutes, while making the dumplings.

Making the Dumpling Batter
Make the dumpling batter by sifting together flour, baking powder, xanthan gum and salt in a medium bowl. Add chopped chives or other fresh herbs. Add melted butter, milk and egg to the dry ingredients.

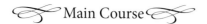

Gently mix with a wooden spoon or fork until mixture is moist and comes together. Do not over-mix or dumplings will be too dense.

Making the Dumplings

Cube the chicken and return to the pot. Add additional broth if mixture is too thick or liquid has cooked down too much. Return to a simmer.

Drop dumpling batter over the surface of the simmering stew by heaping tablespoonfuls. (Note that the dumplings will double in size as they cook.) Cover and simmer until dumplings are cooked through, about 15 minutes. If after 15 minutes they are still not cooked through (use a toothpick or skewer to test), cover pan again and cook for another 5 minutes.

Finishing Up and Serving

Gently stir in peas and parsley. Ladle portions of meat, sauce, vegetables and dumplings into soup plates and serve.

Do not peek while the dumplings are cooking. In order for the dumplings to be light and fluffy, they must steam, not boil. Uncovering the pan releases the steam.

The stew will continue to thicken as it sits.

Each serving contains 624 calories, 10g total fat, 4g saturated fat, 0g trans fat, 133mg cholesterol, 1864mg sodium, 97g carbohydrate, 9g fiber, 11g sugars, 37g protein.

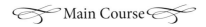

Beth's
Summer Vegetable (Squash) Lasagna
Serves 10

This dish is as colorful as it is flavorful. It can be served warm or at room temperature, making it perfect for summer dining and winter potlucks. This recipe can be made egg-free.*

Ingredients
1 teaspoon salt
15 brown rice or corn lasagna noodles
1 (5-ounce) bag fresh baby spinach
2 tablespoons olive oil, divided
1 large shallot, minced
2 medium zucchini, cut into ⅛-inch thick disks
2 medium yellow squash, cut into ⅛-inch thick disks
Salt and pepper, to taste
2 pounds part-skim ricotta cheese or non-dairy ricotta replacement, divided
4 large eggs*
2 tablespoons dry parsley or 4 tablespoons fresh parsley
4 cups gluten-free marinara sauce, divided
2 cups low-fat mozzarella cheese, shredded, or non-dairy cheese alternative, divided
1 cup grated Parmesan or Romano cheese or non-dairy cheese alternative, divided

Getting Started
In a large pot, bring 6 quarts water to a boil. Stir in 1 teaspoon salt. Add pasta and cook until softened but not fully cooked, about 6 minutes. Rinse with cold water and drain. Lay noodles flat on foil to cool.

Preheat oven to 375°F.

Sautéing the Vegetables
In a large skillet, sauté spinach in 1 tablespoon olive oil just until wilted. Remove from pan and transfer to a plate to cool. Add 1 tablespoon additional oil and sauté minced shallot for 1 minute. Add zucchini and yellow squash and sauté for about 3 minutes or just until squash begins to soften but is not wilted. Add salt and pepper, to taste.

Prevent problem pasta that disintegrates in the pasta water or globs together when refrigerated and reheated by following these tips:
- **Boil in plenty of water.**
  Use at least 4 quarts salted water to cook pasta. Add pasta and return to boil before timing.
- **Always under-cook.**
  Reduce cooking time by 2 to 3 minutes for pasta used in salads. Cut cooking time in half for pasta used in hot sauce and reheated. For lasagna, cook pasta sheets just until soft and pliable.

*For **Egg-Free Vegetable Lasagna,** omit 4 eggs. Combine 4 tablespoons flax meal with 12 tablespoons warm water; let sit 5 minutes until slightly thickened. Then add to recipe to replace 4 eggs.

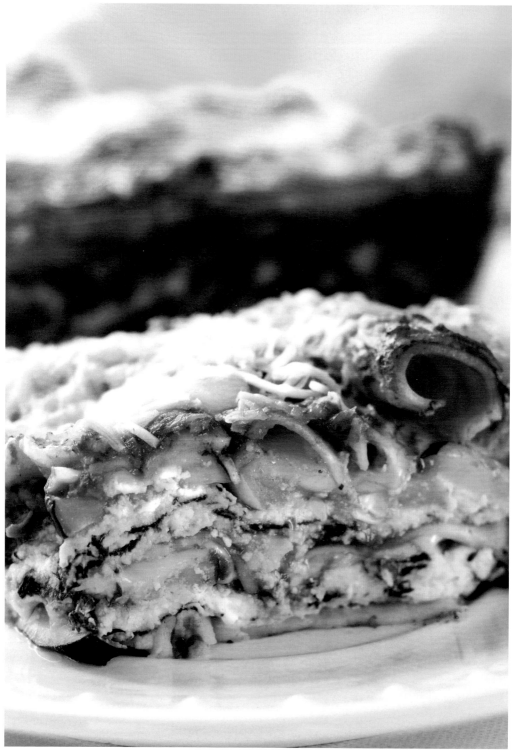

Summer Vegetable (Squash) Lasagna

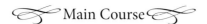

Preparing the Ricotta Mixture
In a small bowl, combine ricotta cheese, eggs and parsley. Add spinach and mix well.

Putting It Together
Spread a small amount of marinara sauce in the bottom of a 9x13-inch pan with a 2-inch high rim.

Arrange 4 noodles lengthwise over sauce and 1 across the bottom, overlapping edges. Spread half the ricotta mixture over the pasta. Arrange half the squash over the top. Sprinkle with ¾ cup mozzarella and ½ cup Parmesan cheese.

Top with another layer of lasagna noodles followed by half the remaining pasta sauce.

Top with remaining ricotta mixture, squash and ¾ cup mozzarella.

Top with remaining lasagna noodles. Spoon remaining marinara sauce over the pasta.

To the Oven and Done
Cover lasagna loosely with aluminum foil. Set on a baking sheet and bake in preheated oven 30 minutes.

Remove foil and top with remaining mozzarella and Parmesan cheese.

Bake uncovered 30 minutes or until hot and bubbly.

Let stand 10 minutes before serving or serve at room temperature.

To store cooked pasta, rinse it in cold water and drain well. Toss with 1 to 2 tablespoons olive oil and cool completely. Refrigerate in a covered container and use within 1 day for cold dishes, 3 days for hot.

For best results, choose corn pasta or quinoa pasta. Rice pasta can become brittle and dry when refrigerated overnight.

Each serving contains 514 calories, 23g total fat, 11g saturated fat, 0g trans fat, 138mg cholesterol, 882mg sodium, 50g carbohydrate, 5g fiber, 28g protein.

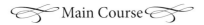 Main Course

Beth's
Maple Cider Vinegar Glazed Roasted Turkey
Makes one 10- to 16-pound bird

Low and slow are the secrets to making this turkey. Roasting at 325°F produces a beautiful golden-brown outside and juicy, succulent meat inside. Squash and Cranberry Sage Stuffing (page 134) can be cooked in the bird with extra baked separately. Serve with Mushroom Gravy on page 139, if desired.

Ingredients
1 (10-16 pound) fresh or frozen turkey

Rub
Makes 6 tablespoons
2 tablespoons light brown sugar
2 tablespoons coarse sea salt (less if watching sodium intake)
1 teaspoon poultry seasoning
½ teaspoon ground mustard
½ teaspoon garlic powder
½ teaspoon paprika
½ teaspoon ground cinnamon

Glaze
3 tablespoons pure maple syrup
3 tablespoons olive oil
3 tablespoons cider vinegar

Making the Rub
Prepare Rub by combining brown sugar and seasonings. Spread Rub over entire turkey and into cavities. Set bird in roasting pan. Cover with plastic wrap and let sit, refrigerated, overnight.

Getting Started
Preheat oven to 325°F.

Making the Stuffing
Prepare Squash and Cranberry Sage Stuffing (page 134) or use your favorite stuffing recipe.

Stuffing the Bird
Stuff turkey loosely with stuffing. Truss bird or cover stuffed cavities with aluminum foil to prevent burning.

Turkey giblets are a flavorful addition to gravy and stuffing. Remove them from the bird and rinse well. Simmer them in 1½ cups water with salt, carrot pieces, onion and parsley until they're tender. (Add more water, as needed.) Remove giblets, cool and chop. Reserve liquid to use in your gravy.

To thaw a frozen turkey, place it in the refrigerator, about 24 hours for every 5 pounds (a 15-pound bird needs 3 days). Alternatively, thaw your bird in a cold-water bath, about 30 minutes per pound (7½ hours for a 15-pound turkey). Refrigerate thawed bird until ready to roast.

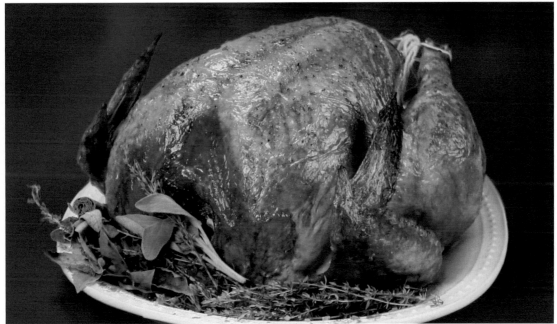

Maple Cider Vinegar Glazed Roasted Turkey

Making the Glaze
Combine maple syrup, olive oil and cider vinegar. Brush over turkey.

Finishing Up—To the Oven and Out
Set turkey in preheated oven and bake 3 to 3½ hours, basting* frequently, until a meat thermometer registers 165°F in the thickest part of the thigh.

Remove turkey from the oven and let stand 20 minutes before carving. Remove stuffing, if used, to a serving dish and slice turkey.

Each 4-ounce serving of white meat (without skin) contains 153 calories, 1g total fat, 0g saturated fat, 0g trans fat, 94mg cholesterol, 59mg sodium, 0g carbohydrate, 0g fiber, 34g protein.

Each 4-ounce serving of dark meat (without skin) contains 183 calories, 5g total fat, 2g saturated fat, 0g trans fat, 127mg cholesterol, 89mg sodium, 0g carbohydrate, 0g fiber, 33g protein.

MORE TURKEY TIPS
Dressed and Ready Never stuff your bird ahead of time. It should be stuffed just before it's put in the oven. Stuffing the turkey increases its cooking time by 5 to 7 minutes per pound. Check the temperature of the stuffing before removing the turkey from the oven. Stuffing must register at least 160°F before it's safe to eat.

Trussed Turkey For a prettier presentation, wind kitchen twine around the legs of your turkey and tuck drumsticks close to the bird's cavity. If you stuff your turkey, trussing keeps the stuffing moist. Another way to prevent stuffing from drying out is to cover the cavity with aluminum foil.

Roasting times vary depending on the size of the turkey. A stuffed turkey must bake 30 to 60 minutes longer than an unstuffed bird.

*Baste turkey with gluten-free chicken broth the first few times until enough juices collect in the pan for basting.

Roast an unstuffed turkey at 325°F, 15 minutes for every pound. A 15-pound turkey requires 3 hours and 45 minutes. If skin browns too quickly, cover the bird loosely with foil.

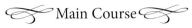

Beth's
Chicken Enchiladas with Peaches, Black Beans and Tomato Chipotle Sauce
Serves 4

A great make-ahead recipe, these enchiladas are ideal for a buffet, potluck or family dinner. This dish is moderately hot but not ear-burning. (Chipotle pepper gives it a little kick.) Adjust the fire by cutting the amount of chipotle powder in half, or to taste.

Ingredients
3 boneless, skinless chicken breast halves (1-1¼ pounds, total)
2 teaspoons olive oil
Salt and pepper, to taste
1 cup shredded sharp cheddar cheese or non-dairy cheese alternative, more for topping, optional
8 gluten-free flour tortillas or 12 gluten-free corn tortillas*

Filling
2 tablespoons olive oil
1 large shallot, minced
2 cloves garlic, minced
¼ teaspoon ground chipotle pepper, or to taste
1 (4½-ounce) can chopped mild green chilis, drained
Juice of half a lime
3 fresh peaches, pitted and chopped, or frozen peach slices, thawed and chopped
1 cup canned black beans, rinsed and drained

Tomato Chipotle Sauce
1 tablespoon olive oil
1 small onion, chopped
3 cloves garlic, chopped
2 pounds ripe plum tomatoes, cored and chopped, or 1 (28-ounce) can diced tomatoes, drained
½-1 teaspoon ground chipotle pepper, or to taste
½ cup gluten-free, dairy-free chicken broth
½ cup sour cream or non-dairy sour cream alternative

Getting Started
Preheat oven to 375°F.
Line a baking pan with foil or parchment. Set chicken breasts in the

*If using corn tortillas, wrap them in a moist paper towel and microwave for 30 seconds to soften. Handle quickly to prevent tortillas from becoming brittle.

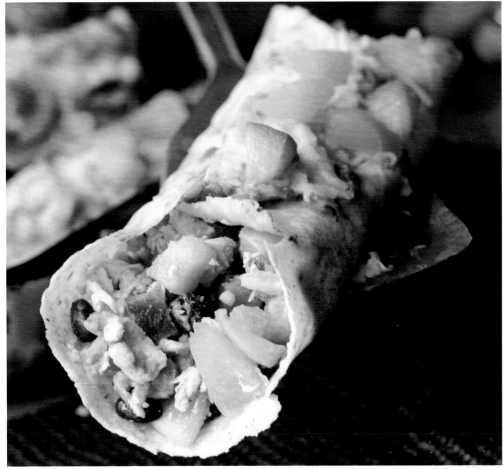

Chicken Enchiladas with Peaches, Black Beans and Tomato Chipotle Sauce

prepared pan and drizzle with 2 teaspoons olive oil. Sprinkle with salt and pepper, to taste.

Baking the Chicken
Place chicken in preheated oven and bake 20 minutes or just until juices run clear. Remove from oven and cool. When cool enough to handle, finely chop the chicken and set aside.

Lower oven temperature to 350°F. Lightly oil a 9x13x2-inch baking pan.

Making the Filling
To make filling, heat 2 tablespoons oil in a skillet over low-medium heat and sauté shallot and garlic until soft, about 3 minutes. Add chopped chicken and stir to coat with mixture. Sprinkle ¼ teaspoon ground chipotle over chicken and sauté about 30 seconds. Add chilis and lime

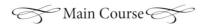

juice and saute 3 minutes. Add peaches and black beans and stir to warm. Remove from heat and set aside while making the sauce.

Making the Sauce

To make the sauce, heat 1 tablespoon olive oil in a medium saucepan. Add onion and garlic and sauté to soften. Add tomatoes and sauté briefly. Add chipotle pepper and sauté an additional 30 seconds. Add chicken broth. Cover and simmer about 15 minutes (5 minutes if using canned tomatoes) or until tomatoes begin to fall apart. Purée mixture in a blender or use an immersion blender. If mixture becomes too thick, add more chicken broth. Stir in sour cream.

Putting It Together

Set 1 tortilla in prepared baking pan and spoon 1 tablespoon sauce over the tortilla. Place a generous scoop of filling (⅓ to ½ cup) in a line across the tortilla just above the center. Sprinkle with shredded cheese, if desired. Roll the tortilla tightly and nestle it against the edge of the pan so it won't unravel. Repeat until all tortillas and filling are used. Spoon remaining sauce over the enchiladas and sprinkle with additional cheese, if desired.

Finishing Up

Cover pan with lightly oiled aluminum foil. Place enchiladas in preheated oven and bake 20 minutes or until tortillas are soft and warmed through. Serve with extra cheese, if desired.

Each serving contains 706 calories, 32g total fat, 12g saturated fat, 0g trans fat, 96mg cholesterol, 778mg sodium, 71g carbohydrate, 14g fiber, 40g protein.

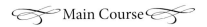

Braised Beef Short Ribs
Serves 4
(RECIPE BY MATTHEW KADEY)

Braising produces fall-off-the-bone tender meat with an immensely rich sauce. Four 1-pound lamb shanks can be used instead of beef short ribs, if desired.

Ingredients
4 pounds lean beef short ribs
Salt and pepper, to taste
1 tablespoon vegetable oil
1 large onion, diced
3 garlic cloves, chopped
1 cup dry red wine
8 plum tomatoes
1 tablespoon tomato paste
1 tablespoon dried sage or thyme
1 teaspoon ground cumin
½ teaspoon fennel seeds
¼ teaspoon salt
¼ teaspoon freshly ground black pepper
Cilantro or parsley, for garnish

Getting Started
Preheat oven to 300°F.

Rinse short ribs. Pat dry with a paper towel and season with salt and pepper.

Braising the Ribs
Heat 1 tablespoon oil in a large ovenproof Dutch oven over medium-high heat. Brown meat on all sides, in batches if necessary. Remove meat from pan.

Making the Tomato Mixture
Add onions and garlic to pan and cook for 3 minutes. Add wine, bring to a boil and simmer until reduced by half, about 5 to 8 minutes.

In a blender or food processor, purée together tomatoes, tomato paste, sage, cumin, fennel, salt and pepper. Add tomato mixture to pan, along with meat.

Into the Oven and Out
Cover pan and cook in preheated oven for 2½ hours or until very tender. Flip meat once halfway through cooking.

Place meat on serving plate. Ladle sauce over top and garnish with fresh herbs.

Each serving contains 470 calories, 26g total fat, 10g saturated fat, 0g trans fat, 113mg cholesterol, 229mg sodium, 10g carbohydrate, 2g fiber, 39g protein.

Crown Pork Roast with Apple Cranberry Stuffing
Serves 6 to 8
(RECIPE BY ROB LANDOLPHI)

A crown roast is a pork rib roast that's "Frenched," i.e., the meat is removed from the bone tips. It's tied into a crown formation, seasoned, stuffed and roasted. The presentation is as elegant as it is delicious—juicy, flavorful meat mingles with tasty bread stuffing.

Ingredients
1 tablespoon fresh rosemary, finely chopped
3 teaspoons salt, divided
1¼ teaspoons freshly ground black pepper, divided
1 (8-pound) crown pork roast
8 cups gluten-free whole-grain bread, lightly toasted and cubed
2 Granny Smith apples, cored, peeled and finely chopped
½ cup butter or non-dairy alternative
1 cup diced onions

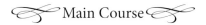

2 cups diced celery
2 cups fresh cranberries
½ cup sugar
¼ cup apple juice
¼ cup gluten-free, dairy-free chicken broth
1 teaspoon poultry seasoning

Getting Started
Preheat oven to 375°F.

Preparing the Roast
In a small bowl, combine rosemary, 2 teaspoons salt and 1 teaspoon pepper. Rub entire roast thoroughly with rosemary mixture. Place pork roast in roasting pan, rib tips up.

Making the Stuffing
Place bread cubes and apples in large bowl and set aside.

In a large skillet, melt butter over medium heat and sauté onions and celery until tender, about 10 minutes. Add cranberries and sugar, cooking until cranberries burst, about 3 to 4 minutes.

Add cranberry mixture to bread mixture and stir in apple juice, chicken broth, 1 teaspoon salt, ¼ teaspoon black pepper and poultry seasoning. Mix until just blended.

Stuffing and Baking the Roast
Loosely fill the cavity of the pork roast with apple cranberry stuffing. (Spoon extra stuffing into a greased oven-proof dish and place in the oven 30 minutes before the roast is done.) Cover the stuffing and tips of the rib bones with foil. Place in preheated oven and bake 2 hours.

Remove foil and cook another 30 to 40 minutes, until stuffing browns slightly on top

and internal temperature of pork reads 150°F on a meat thermometer.

Out of the Oven and Serving
Remove from oven and allow to rest 20 minutes before serving. After presenting at the dinner table, stuffing can be removed and placed in a bowl. Using a sharp knife, cut the roast into 1-rib servings.

Each 1-rib serving with stuffing contains 540 calories, 17g total fat, 5g saturated fat, 0g trans fat, 132mg cholesterol, 743mg sodium, 42g carbohydrate, 2g fiber, 52g protein.

Ask your butcher to trim and prepare the crown roast for you.

Honey Glazed Pork Tenderloin with Maple Mashed Sweet Potatoes
Serves 4
(RECIPE BY MATTHEW KADEY)

Low-fat, inexpensive pork tenderloin takes perfectly to this honey-infused glaze. Extra tenderloin can be sliced and served cold in salads and sandwiches. Butternut squash works well as a substitute for sweet potatoes, if desired.

Ingredients
2 pork tenderloins (about 1½ pounds total), excess fat removed
Salt and pepper, to taste
2 tablespoons vegetable oil, divided
2 tablespoons honey
2 tablespoons gluten-free soy sauce*
1 tablespoon rice vinegar
½ teaspoon hot sauce, optional
2 garlic cloves, grated
1 (1-inch) piece ginger, grated

Maple Mashed Sweet Potatoes
1½ pounds sweet potatoes, peeled and diced

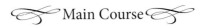

3 tablespoons milk or unflavored non-dairy
milk alternative
2 tablespoons pure maple syrup
1 tablespoon butter or non-dairy alternative
1 (1-inch) piece ginger, grated
¼ teaspoon ground nutmeg
Salt, to taste

Getting Started
Preheat oven to 425°F

Prepping the Pork
Season pork with salt and pepper. In an oven-proof skillet, heat 1 tablespoon oil over medium-high heat. Add pork and sear all sides until golden brown, about 5 minutes.

Making the Glaze
To make honey glaze, combine 1 tablespoon vegetable oil, honey, soy sauce, rice vinegar, hot sauce, garlic and ginger in a bowl.

Transfer half the honey mixture to a separate bowl and set aside.

To the Oven and Out
Spread half the glaze over pork and transfer skillet to preheated oven. Roast pork until a thermometer inserted into thickest part of meat registers 145°F, about 15 minutes. Coat with remaining glaze and let rest 5 to 10 minutes before slicing.

Making the Potatoes
As pork cooks, steam sweet potatoes until very tender. With a potato masher or in a food processor, mash together potatoes, milk, maple syrup, butter, ginger, nutmeg and salt.

Serving the Meal
Serve mashed sweet potatoes with pork slices.

Each serving contains 663 calories, 17g total fat, 10g saturated fat, 0g trans fat, 169mg cholesterol, 1338mg sodium, 52g carbohydrate, 5g fiber, 72g protein.

*Can't have soy? Replace soy sauce with gluten-free coconut aminos, available from Coconut Secret (coconutsecret.com). For other gluten-free or allergy-friendly products, see Shopping List, page 189.

Mango Chicken Curry
Serves 4
(RECIPE BY MATTHEW KADEY)

Mango and chicken are a wonderful flavor combination and come together beautifully in this sweet curry. Using store-bought curry powder is a time-saving step that still produces delicious curry.

Ingredients
1 tablespoon coconut oil or oil of choice
1 large onion, chopped
1 red bell pepper, chopped
3 garlic cloves, minced
2 tablespoons fresh minced ginger
1½ tablespoons curry powder
1 teaspoon cumin seeds
¼ teaspoon cayenne powder
2 tablespoons cider vinegar or
white vinegar
1¼ cups gluten-free, dairy-free chicken broth
2 cups diced mango, fresh or frozen, divided
¼ teaspoon salt
¼ teaspoon freshly ground black pepper
1½ pounds skinless, boneless chicken thighs,
cut into 1-inch pieces
⅓ cup golden raisins
Juice of ½ lemon
½ cup canned coconut milk
4 cups cooked brown rice
¼ cup chopped cilantro, for garnish

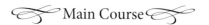

Getting Started
Heat oil in a large skillet over medium heat.

Making the Curry
Add onions and cook, stirring occasionally, until softened, about 5 minutes.

Add red bell pepper; cook 2 minutes.

Add garlic, ginger, curry powder, cumin seeds and cayenne; cook 1 minute.

Add vinegar, broth, 1 cup mango, salt and pepper to the skillet.

Bring to a boil, lower heat and simmer for 15 minutes, stirring occasionally.

Blending it Together
Carefully place the contents of the skillet into a blender or food processor container and blend until smooth.

Finishing Up
Return the sauce to the skillet and add chicken pieces and raisins. Return to a simmer and cook covered for 8 to 10 minutes, or until chicken is cooked through.

Add remaining mango pieces, lemon juice and coconut milk; heat 2 minutes.

Serve curry over cooked brown rice and garnish with cilantro.

Each serving contains 646 calories, 19g total fat, 10g saturated fat, 0g trans fat, 139mg cholesterol, 604mg sodium, 80g carbohydrate, 8g fiber, 25g sugars, 41g protein.

> For convenience, use frozen cubed mango in this recipe. It's often located alongside the frozen berries in supermarkets. No need to thaw the cubes first.

> Chicken thighs will provide more flavor than breast meat and cost less.

Pork Carnitas with Citrus Sauce
Serves 6
(RECIPE BY MARY CAPONE)

A Southwest menu is not complete without tender pork carnitas. This recipe combines the sweet taste of orange with the savory flavor of pork. For a main course, add a side of chopped onions, avocado, tomatoes and your favorite salsa.

Ingredients
1 pound boneless country-style pork ribs or pork loin chops, cut into 1-inch cubes
5 cloves garlic, smashed
½ teaspoon ground cinnamon
1½ cups orange juice
1 tablespoon orange zest
2 cups water
1½ teaspoons sea salt

Cooking the Pork
In large skillet, add all ingredients. Bring to boil uncovered. Reduce heat and cover, simmering for 1½ hours or until pork is tender and comes apart easily with a fork. Stir occasionally, turning meat over halfway through cooking. Add more water if needed to keep meat partly covered in liquid.

Uncover and let liquid reduce, about 15 minutes.

Finishing Up
Remove meat to cutting board. Using a fork and knife, shred into small pieces. Return meat to pan to absorb the last of the sauce. Serve on warm corn tortillas.

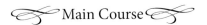
Each serving contains 193 calories, 11g total fat, 4g saturated fat, 0g trans fat, 45mg cholesterol, 614mg sodium, 8g carbohydrate, 0g fiber, 16g protein.

Roast Leg of Lamb with Garlic Herb Crust and Gravy
Serves 6 to 8
(RECIPE BY SUESON VESS)

High in zinc and B vitamins, lamb is traditional Easter fare and is a treat any time of year.

Ingredients
1 bone-in leg of lamb (about 6 pounds)
3 sprigs fresh rosemary
4-5 cloves garlic or 1 shallot
1 teaspoon olive oil
½ teaspoon each sea salt and pepper
4-6 cups gluten-free, dairy-free beef or lamb broth, divided
2-3 tablespoons arrowroot powder or cornstarch

Getting Started
Preheat oven to 400°F. Place lamb on roasting rack in roasting pan.

Preparing the Spices and Meat
Remove the leaves from the rosemary sprigs. Add rosemary and garlic to food processor fitted with knife blade and blend.

Rub lamb with olive oil. Sprinkle with salt and pepper. Pat rosemary and garlic blend on all sides of lamb. Pour 1 cup beef or lamb broth in the bottom of the roasting pan.

To the Oven and Out:
Place pan in preheated oven and cook for 30 minutes. Reduce heat to 325°F. Check internal temperature of roast after 1 hour and baste with pan drippings. Meat is done when meat thermometer registers 145°F for medium rare, 155°F to 160°F for medium, 165°F to 170°F for well done.

Take lamb from oven, remove from pan and set aside while making gravy.

Making the Gravy
Use broth to deglaze roasting pan and loosen browned bits of meat. Strain liquid to remove tough bits. Make a slurry by combining ¼ cup cold water with arrowroot, stirring until dissolved. Pour slurry into pan with deglazed liquid and continue to stir over medium-low heat until desired thickness. Add additional arrowroot slurry if needed. Taste and adjust seasoning.

Finishing Up
Allow lamb to rest for 10 to 15 minutes. Then slice and serve with hot gravy.

Each 3-ounce serving contains 155 calories, 5g total fat, 2g saturated fat, 0g trans fat, 78mg cholesterol, 231mg sodium, 2g carbohydrate, 0g fiber, 23g protein.

The key to delicious gravy is a flavorful broth. Prepare homemade beef or lamb broth up to 3 months in advance and freeze until ready to use. If using store-bought broth, enhance flavor by simmering it with a diced onion and carrots while lamb roasts. Read the label carefully to be sure the broth is gluten free.

Pasture-raised, grass-fed lamb is lower in fat and higher in omega 3 fatty acids. Find grass-fed meat at your local supermarket or visit eatwild.com and grassfedtraditions.com.

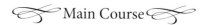

Sloppy Joe Kid-Wich
Makes 10 to 12 mini sandwiches
(RECIPE BY SUESON VESS)

Enjoy this meaty recipe on gluten-free mini-buns, perfect party fare for kids and adults. This recipe can be prepared in advance and refrigerated for 2 days. It freezes well; reheat before serving.

Ingredients
1 teaspoon olive oil
1 cup chopped onion
1 cup chopped sweet bell peppers
1 pound ground beef or turkey
1 teaspoon ground turmeric
½ teaspoon crushed chili flakes, more or less to taste
¼ teaspoon ground cloves
2 tablespoons cider vinegar
1 (7-ounce) jar tomato paste, low/no salt added
2 tablespoons honey
¼-½ cup water

Sautéing
In a large skillet, heat olive oil and sauté onions and peppers over medium heat until softened.

Add ground meat, turmeric, chili flakes and cloves and cook until no pink color remains in meat, about 5 to 7 minutes.

Simmering
Add cider vinegar, tomato paste, honey and water, ¼ cup at a time until desired consistency. Stir to combine.

Simmer uncovered for 10 minutes. Taste and adjust seasoning. Serve hot.

Each serving contains 107 calories, 5g total fat, 2g saturated fat, 0g trans fat, 23mg cholesterol, 43mg sodium, 8g carbohydrate, 1g fiber, 8g protein.

Sunchoke Bacon Pasta
Serves 6
(RECIPE BY MATTHEW KADEY)

Canadian bacon is signficantly leaner than regular bacon, making it a healthier way to add meaty texture to pasta dishes. The thinner you slice the sunchokes, the quicker they will cook.

Ingredients
16 ounces gluten-free pasta, such as penne or fusilli
1 tablespoon canola or light olive oil
6 slices (about ½ pound) Canadian bacon, chopped
1 pound sunchokes, scrubbed and thinly sliced
1 bunch fresh flat-leaf parsley, roughly chopped
3 tablespoons extra virgin olive oil
Juice of ½ lemon
½ teaspoon red chili flakes
¼ teaspoon sea salt
¼ teaspoon freshly ground black pepper
Parmesan cheese or non-dairy alternative, optional

Making the Pasta
In a large pot of salted water, prepare pasta according to package directions.

Cooking the Bacon and Sunchokes
Meanwhile, heat oil in a large skillet over medium heat. Cook bacon until cooked through, about 5 minutes. Remove bacon from skillet and place on a paper towel to drain. Add sunchokes to skillet and cook until browned and softened, about 10 minutes.

Putting It Together
Drain pasta, return to pot and stir in bacon, sunchokes and parsley.

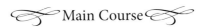

Making the Dressing

In a small bowl, whisk together olive oil, lemon juice, chili flakes, salt and black pepper.

Finishing Up

Stir olive oil mixture into the pasta mixture. Top with grated Parmesan cheese, if desired.

Each serving contains 443 calories, 11g total fat, 2g saturated fat, 0g trans fat, 18mg cholesterol, 470mg sodium, 78g carbohydrate, 6g fiber, 11g protein.

Spiced Steak with Island Barbecue Sauce
Serves 4
(RECIPE BY MARY CAPONE)

Simple spices and a fruity sauce transform a less expensive cut of steak into a dish fit for royalty.

Ingredients
1½ pounds tri-tip steak
2 tablespoons coarse sea salt
½ tablespoon pink
or black peppercorns, crushed
1 teaspoon grated fresh ginger
1 tablespoon brown sugar

Getting Started

Pat meat dry with a paper towel. Place meat in a pan.

Spicing the Meat

Mix spices and sugar together in a bowl. Rub spice mix onto both sides of the meat, pressing spices gently into the flesh. Refrigerate meat for at least 1 hour. Remove meat from refrigerator and brush top side with half the Island Barbecue Sauce.

Grilling the Meat

Place top side down on slightly greased hot grill. Brush remaining barbecue sauce on reverse side.

Cook steak for 8 minutes per side for medium to medium-rare.

Finishing Up

Remove meat and let rest for 5 minutes before slicing. For best results, cut meat in thin slices against the grain at a 45° angle.

Island Barbecue Sauce
Makes about 1 cup
½ cup ketchup
1 tablespoon orange juice
2 teaspoons minced fresh ginger root
1 clove garlic, minced
2 teaspoons dark blackstrap molasses
1 teaspoon balsamic vinegar
1 teaspoon gluten-free soy sauce
½ lime, juiced
Salt and pepper, to taste

Making the Sauce

Combine ingredients together. Refrigerate until used.

Each serving of steak with barbecue sauce contains 340 calories, 15g total fat, 5g saturated fat, 0g trans fat, 109mg cholesterol, 1666mg sodium, 16g carbohydrate, 1g fiber, 36g protein.

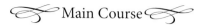
Three-Bean Vegetarian Chili
Makes 10 cups
(RECIPE BY REBECCA REILLY)

Serve this with gluten-free corn bread, polenta or brown basmati rice for a satisfying meal.

Ingredients

3 tablespoons extra-virgin olive oil
1 large onion, coarsely chopped
1 tablespoon chopped fresh garlic
2 stalks celery, coarsely chopped
3 carrots, chopped diagonally
1 green pepper, diced
1 red pepper, diced
1 tablespoon chili powder
2-3 teaspoons ground cumin
2 teaspoons dried oregano
½-1 teaspoon salt
1 (4-ounce) can chopped green chili peppers, drained
1 (12-ounce) package gluten-free tempeh
1 (35-ounce) can whole peeled tomatoes with juice, chopped coarsely
2 cups tomato puree
24 grinds fresh black pepper
1 (15-ounce) can kidney beans, rinsed and drained
1 (15-ounce) can garbanzo beans, rinsed and drained
1 (15-ounce) can black beans, rinsed and drained

Sautéing

Heat olive oil in a large pot and sauté onion and garlic until translucent.

Toss in celery, carrots, peppers and chili powder and stir for 1 minute.

Finishing Up

Add remaining ingredients and cook until carrots are tender. Adjust seasonings to taste. Serve hot.

Each serving contains 289 calories, 9g total fat, 2g saturated fat, 0g trans fat, 0mg cholesterol, 41g carbohydrate, 812mg sodium, 11g fiber, 16g protein.

SIDES, SALADS
&
SAUCES

"The right sides, salads and sauces turn ordinary meals into extraordinary spreads."

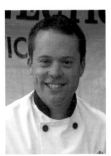

Recipes by
Robert Landolphi
and other celebrity chefs

Robert Landolphi

Hampton, Connecticut

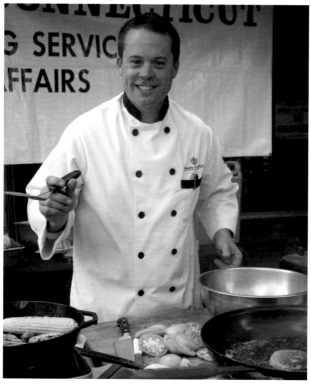

"Empty your mind of preconceived notions that gluten-free food can't taste good."

A s a graduate of Johnson & Wales University, my culinary training focused on techniques and methods that could turn every meal into something flavorful, memorable and unique.

I worked in food service management for many years and had my own bakery on the edge of the University of Connecticut campus. But my career made a 180° turn when my wife Angela developed celiac disease and was forced to go gluten free.

With her diagnosis, I had to reinvent all those years of training in order to make our meals suit her dietary needs. I could no longer thicken gravy with a roux of flour and butter or make my signature fried onion rings with wheat flour. I even had to watch the ingredients that went into my salads— no croutons, no soy sauce dressing, no crunchy noodles.

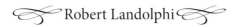

I found out early on that gluten-free ingredients behave differently than their wheat-filled counterparts. At first, my cookies spread when I wanted them to rise. My breads were like doorstops. The gravy I made for our first gluten-free Thanksgiving separated after a couple of hours.

I spent hours becoming familiar with the nuances of my new ingredients, finding the right ones and the flour blends that would create the correct flavors and textures and give the best results. I made so many mistakes at first but I couldn't afford to be afraid of failure. My family was waiting for dinner! For their sake, I threw away all my wheat flour-based notions and relearned new principles of food chemistry. Little by little, the results got better.

Perhaps if Angela had never been diagnosed with celiac disease, I would not know about the wonders of quinoa or that my signature onion rings would be even lighter when fried in a batter of rice flour.

Now I tell anyone who is starting the gluten-free diet: "Empty your pantry of all those wheat- and gluten-based products and your mind of any preconceived notions that gluten-free food can't taste good. Get ready for a delicious culinary adventure!"

A graduate of Johnson & Wales University College of Culinary Arts, Robert Landolphi is culinary operations manager at the University of Connecticut where he has set up separate dining facilities and menus for gluten-free students. He educates audiences around the country with his gluten-free cooking classes. When he's not developing innovative, gluten-free recipes, Landolphi writes for a variety of print media and conducts regular radio and TV interviews around the nation.

Landolphi is author of *Gluten Free Every Day Cookbook* and *Quick-Fix Gluten Free* (Andrews McMeel Publishing, LLC).

Where to find Robert Landolphi:
glutenfreechefrob.com

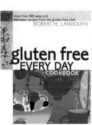

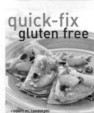

These books are available at LivingWithout.com.

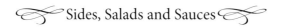

SIDES, SALADS AND SAUCES

Rob's
Butternut Squash Patties with Honey Citrus Arugula Salad

Serves 6

This was created for an event in Connecticut to raise money for farmland preservation. A vegetable lover's delight, it's brimming with healthy butternut squash, carrots and red onions and topped with a sweet tangy dressing and peppery arugula. This recipe can be made egg-free.*

Ingredients
1 cup diced red onion
5 tablespoons olive oil, divided
2 cups peeled, seeded and grated butternut squash
½ cup peeled and grated carrot
¼ cup diced scallions
2 tablespoons honey
1 large egg,* beaten
¼ cup chickpea flour
2 tablespoons gluten-free bread crumbs
¼ teaspoon ground cinnamon
⅛ teaspoon ground chipotle pepper
⅛ teaspoon salt
3 cups baby arugula
Honey Citrus Dressing
2 ounces feta cheese, crumbled, optional

Getting Started
In medium skillet, cook onion in 1 tablespoon olive oil over medium-high heat until softened. Set aside.

Mixing the Ingredients
Place grated butternut squash in large bowl with grated carrot, scallions,

*For **Egg-Free Patties,** omit 1 egg. Combine 1 tablespoon flax meal with 3 tablespoons warm water. Let sit for 5 minutes until slightly thickened. Combine flax meal mixture with other ingredients to make patties.

Baby spinach, watercress and mesclun greens are tasty substitutes for arugula.

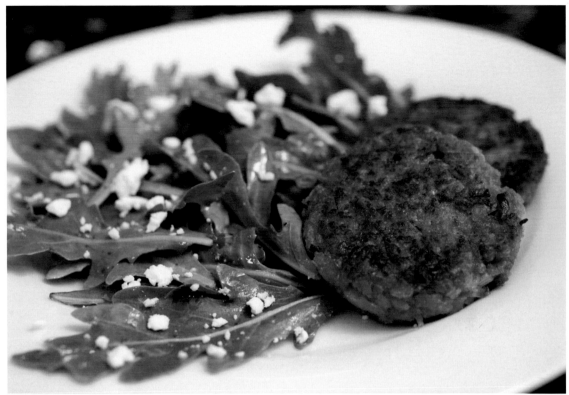

Butternut Squash Patties with Honey Citrus Arugula Salad

cooked red onion, honey, egg, chickpea flour, bread crumbs, cinnamon, chipotle pepper, and salt.

Mix all ingredients together in bowl, and refrigerate 30 minutes. If mixture is wet, add extra gluten-free bread crumbs.

Making the Patties
Heat 4 tablespoons olive oil in a large skillet over medium-high heat. Working in batches, make ¼-cup size patties and place in skillet. Fry patties until golden brown, 3 minutes per side, adding more olive oil as needed, until all patties are cooked.

Place cooked patties on a sheet pan and keep in a warm oven while making the salad.

Making the Salad
Place arugula in a large bowl and toss with just enough Honey Citrus Dressing to lightly coat greens. Place hot patties on a platter, top with dressed arugula and sprinkle with feta cheese, if desired.

Always make sure the greens are completely dry before tossing with dressing. Go lightly on the dressing, as too much will result in a soggy salad.

Honey Citrus Dressing

Makes ¾ cup

Ingredients

2 tablespoons honey
¼ cup lemon juice
½ teaspoon Dijon mustard
½ cup olive oil
Salt, to taste
Freshly ground black pepper, to taste

Salad dressing can be made ahead and stored in the refrigerator in an airtight container for up to 1 week. Bring it back to room temperature and re-whisk to emulsify it before dressing the salad.

Making the Dressing

In a blender, blend together honey, lemon juice and Dijon mustard. With blender running on low, slowly drizzle in olive oil until dressing is thoroughly blended. Season to taste with salt and pepper.

Each serving contains 379 calories, 32g total fat, 5g saturated fat, 0g trans fat, 35mg cholesterol, 90mg sodium, 26g carbohydrate, 2g fiber, 15g sugars, 3g protein.

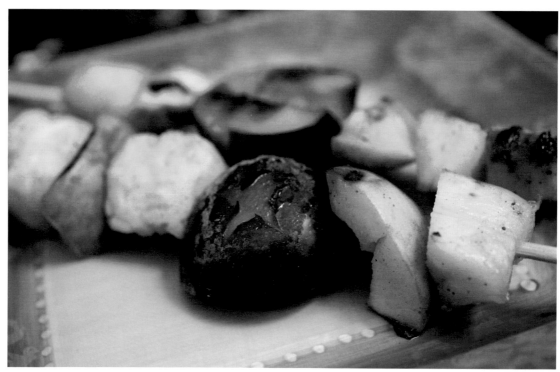

Maple Glazed Fruit Skewers

Rob's
Maple Glazed Fruit Skewers
Serves 4

This is one of my favorite sides for Sunday brunch. These skewered chunks of pineapple, peaches, plums and nectarines are bursting with the flavors of maple syrup, vanilla and cinnamon.

Ingredients
½ cup pure maple syrup
1 teaspoon pure vanilla extract
¼ teaspoon ground nutmeg
⅛ teaspoon ground cinnamon
2 firm peaches, halved and pitted
2 firm plums, halved and pitted
2 firm nectarines, halved and pitted
1 cup pineapple chunks
4 wooden skewers, soaked in water 20 minutes
1 pint non-dairy vanilla yogurt

Making the Glaze
In a medium bowl, whisk together maple syrup, vanilla, nutmeg and cinnamon. Add the fruit and toss gently to coat with glaze. Refrigerate for at least 1 hour.

Getting Ready to Grill
Preheat grill to medium-high and generously oil grates. Thread the fruit on the skewers, alternating varieties.

Grilling
Place skewered fruit on the grill cut side down. Cook until heated through and caramelized, 2 to 3 minutes per side.

To the Table
Set on individual plates and serve with a scoop of non-dairy vanilla yogurt.

Each serving contains 312 calories, 3g total fat, 0g saturated fat, 0g trans fat, 0mg cholesterol, 18mg sodium, 70g carbohydrate, 4g fiber, 57g sugars, 5g protein.

Don't feel confined to using just the fruit listed in this recipe. Be creative and mix things up. Apples, pears and under-ripened bananas work well.

Warming spices, such as cinnamon, cloves, ginger and nutmeg, are secret flavor boosters. Bonus: They're virtually calorie-free and studies suggest diets heavy in spices are protective against several chronic diseases.

Rob's
Fried Green Tomato Salad with White Bean Vinaigrette
Serves 6

I always find myself with an abundance of green, unripened tomatoes on the vines just before the fall frost sets in. This is a great way to use them up. Plus it's an attractive-looking salad that will be the talk of any dinner party. This recipe can be made egg-free.*

Ingredients
2 tablespoons extra-virgin olive oil
2 tablespoons white balsamic vinegar
1 tablespoon honey
¼ teaspoon Dijon mustard
1 teaspoon finely chopped fresh parsley
1 clove garlic, minced
⅛ teaspoon salt, plus ½ teaspoon salt
1 (15-ounce) can white beans, drained, rinsed and dried
¼ cup finely diced red bell pepper
1 cup gluten-free yellow cornmeal
2 teaspoons garlic powder
⅛ teaspoon ground chipotle pepper, optional
1 large egg*
1 tablespoon rice milk or milk of choice
Vegetable oil, for frying
4 green tomatoes, cored and sliced ¼-inch thick (24 slices)

Getting Started
In a medium bowl, whisk together the olive oil, vinegar, honey, mustard, parsley, garlic and ⅛ teaspoon of salt. Add the beans and red pepper, tossing to coat thoroughly in the dressing. Set aside.

Preparing the Cornmeal Mixture
In a shallow small bowl, whisk together the cornmeal, garlic powder, remaining ½ teaspoon salt and the chipotle pepper, if using.

Preparing the Egg Mixture
In another shallow bowl, beat together the egg and rice milk.

Frying the Tomatoes
Heat ¼ inch of vegetable oil in a large skillet over medium-high heat. Dip

If you can't find green tomatoes, substitute slices of eggplant or green zucchini.

Chipotle pepper adds a nice spiciness to this dish. For extra heat, add up to ½ teaspoon, to taste.

*For **Egg-Free Green Tomato Salad,** omit 1 egg. Combine 1 tablespoon flax meal with 3 tablespoons warm water. Let sit for 5 minutes until slightly thickened. Combine flax meal mixture with milk.

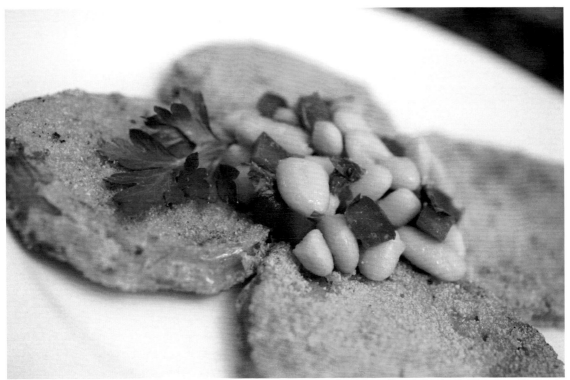

Fried Green Tomato Salad with White Bean Vinaigrette

each tomato slice in the egg mixture. Allow the excess to drip off and dredge both sides in the cornmeal. Fry in the hot oil until golden brown on both sides and then place on paper towels to drain. Continue until all the tomato slices are fried.

Putting It Together
To build each salad, place 4 slices of fried tomatoes on each serving plate and spoon the white bean vinaigrette over the top. Serve immediately. This can also be arranged on 1 large platter for a colorful buffet dish.

Each serving contains 275 calories, 9g total fat, 3g saturated fat, 0g trans fat, 35mg cholesterol, 286mg sodium, 42g carbohydrate, 6g fiber, 9g sugars, 10g protein.

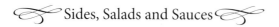

Rob's
Fried Onion Strings with Horseradish Dipping Sauce

Serves 4

Going gluten-free doesn't mean you have to give up yummy onion rings. These are a huge hit with ribs and burgers.

Ingredients
1 cup rice or soy milk
¼ cup gluten-free hot sauce
2 large sweet onions, peeled and sliced in ⅛-inch slices
2 cups white rice flour
1 tablespoon paprika
1 teaspoon salt
2 teaspoons garlic powder
½ teaspoon cayenne pepper
Vegetable oil, for frying

Making the Marinade
In a large bowl, whisk together rice milk and hot sauce. Add onions and allow to marinate at least 1 hour.

Preparing the Flour Mixture
In a shallow bowl, whisk together flour and all the spices.

Getting Ready to Fry
In a large saucepan, heat 3 inches of vegetable oil until a deep–fat thermometer reads 360°F.

Frying the Onion Strings
Remove onions from milk and toss into flour mixture, a handful at a time until completely coated. Add to oil and cook until golden brown, 2 to 3 minutes per batch.

Remove from oil and drain on paper towels. Repeat with remaining onions until all are cooked. Serve with Horseradish Dipping Sauce.

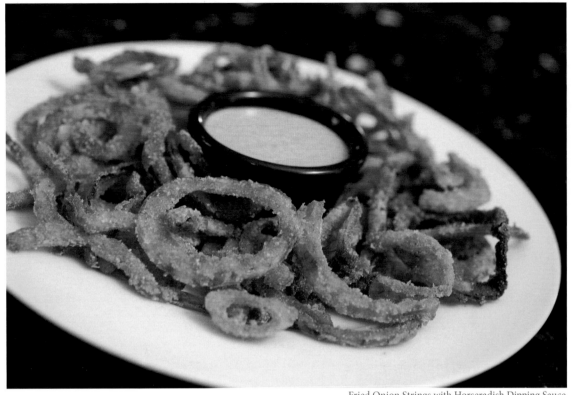

Fried Onion Strings with Horseradish Dipping Sauce

Horseradish Dipping Sauce

Makes ¾ cup

Ingredients

½ cup gluten-free, dairy-free mayonnaise, plain yogurt or
non-dairy alternative
2 tablespoons ketchup
2 tablespoons prepared horseradish
½ teaspoon seasoned salt
⅛ teaspoon cayenne pepper
¼ teaspoon paprika

Making the Dipping Sauce

In small bowl, whisk together all ingredients until incorporated.
Refrigerate in an airtight container until used.

Each serving contains 540 calories, 16g total fat, 2g saturated fat, 0g trans fat,
8mg cholesterol, 1408mg sodium, 94g carbohydrate, 5g fiber, 16g sugars, 7g protein.

Vegenaise, a gluten-free, dairy-free, egg-free mayonnaise, is available from Follow Your Heart (followyourheart.com). For other gluten-free, allergy-friendly products, see Shopping List, page 189.

Rob's
Chimichurri Sauce and Pork Tenderloin
Serves 6

For Chimichurri Sauce with Beef Kebabs, see page 98.

From Argentina, flavorful chimichurri sauce produces show-stopping results when paired with pork tenderloin. Similar to pesto, this powerhouse of flavor makes a tasty marinade or sauce for chicken, beef, pork or even pasta and eggs.

Chimichurri Sauce
Makes 1½ cups

1 cup packed chopped Italian flat leaf parsley
4 cloves garlic, minced
2 tablespoons shallots, minced
1 tablespoon chopped fresh oregano
1½ teaspoons kosher salt
½ teaspoon freshly ground black pepper
½ teaspoon red chili pepper flakes
¾ cup extra virgin olive oil
¼ cup sherry wine vinegar
2 tablespoons lemon juice

Making the Sauce
Place all ingredients in a blender or food processor and pulse until coarsely chopped. Store in an airtight container in the refrigerator until used. This sauce will keep 5 to 7 days in the refrigerator.

Pork Tenderloin
Serves 6
2 pork tenderloins (about 2 pounds)
1 tablespoon olive oil
½ teaspoon kosher salt
½ teaspoon freshly ground black pepper
1½ teaspoons fresh oregano
or ½ teaspoon dried oregano
Chimichurri Sauce

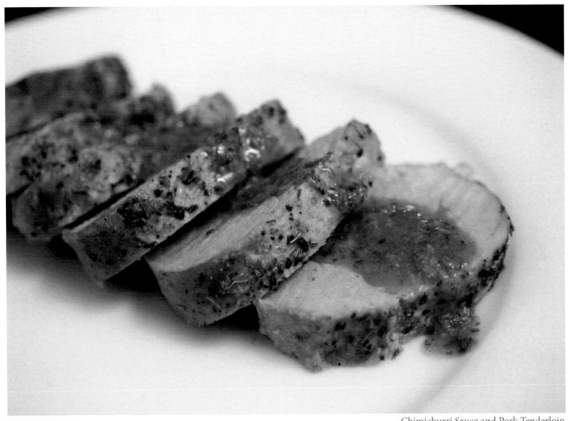

Chimichurri Sauce and Pork Tenderloin

Getting Started
Preheat a grill to medium heat. Rub the pork tenderloin thoroughly with
olive oil and sprinkle with salt, pepper and oregano.

Grilling the Meat
Grill pork for 12 to 15 minutes, turning occasionally, until it reaches 145°F
on an instant-read thermometer.

Finishing Up and Serving
Let the pork rest on a cutting board for 5 minutes before cutting it into
½-inch-thick slices. Place the slices on a platter and spoon Chimichurri
Sauce over the pork just before serving.

Each serving contains 443 calories, 34g total fat, 5g saturated fat, 0g trans fat,
97mg cholesterol, 865mg sodium, 6g carbohydrate, 1g fiber, 0g sugars, 32g protein.

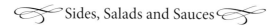
Plum Sauce and Barbecued Chicken Thighs
Serves 8
(RECIPE BY ROBERT LANDOLPHI)

This special sauce is so versatile, it can be transformed into a succulent, mouthwatering, finger-licking barbecue sauce for ribs, burgers or chicken wings or used as it is here to produce flavorful chicken thighs.

Plum Sauce
Makes 2½ cups

½ cup plum jam
½ cup white vinegar
½ cup ketchup
¼ cup honey
2 tablespoons garlic, minced
4 tablespoons lime juice
1 tablespoon minced sweet onion
½ cup plum wine

Making the Plum Sauce
Combine all ingredients (except plum wine) in a saucepan over medium heat until sauce boils. Add plum wine and let sauce simmer 5 minutes before removing from heat. Cool to room temperature.

Ingredients
12 chicken thighs (about 3 pounds)

Dry Rub
3 tablespoons allspice
3 tablespoons brown sugar
3 tablespoons garlic powder
1 tablespoon kosher salt
1 teaspoon ground nutmeg
1 teaspoon ground cinnamon
1 teaspoon dried thyme
1 teaspoon ground mustard

Making the Dry Rub
In a medium mixing bowl, combine all ingredients for dry rub. Stir until thoroughly blended.

Preparing the Chicken
Place chicken thighs in a baking pan. Using hands, massage dry rub mixture over chicken until evenly coated. Cover with plastic wrap and let sit 30 minutes.

Grilling the Meat
Heat the grill to medium heat and grill chicken thighs, skin side down, for 8 to 10 minutes or until golden brown. Turn the chicken over, brush with Plum Sauce, close the lid and cook 5 more minutes until cooked through.

To the Table
Remove from the grill and place chicken on a platter with extra Plum Sauce for dipping.

Each serving contains 230 calories, 3g total fat, 1g saturated fat, 0g trans fat, 51mg cholesterol, 1103mg sodium, 39g carbohydrate, 1g fiber, 30g sugars, 13g protein.

> Plum Sauce can be made ahead and stored in an airtight container in the refrigerator for up to 3 months.

Quinoa Spinach Salad with Mandarin Oranges
Serves 12
(RECIPE BY ROBERT LANDOLPHI)

This trendy and flavorful salad can be served warm as a starter at a dinner party or cold at your neighbor's picnic. It combines quinoa with crisp baby spinach, a sweet maple dressing and a citrusy burst of mandarin oranges.

Ingredients
1 cup white quinoa
1 cup red or black quinoa
4 cups water or gluten-free, dairy-free vegetable broth
6 tablespoons olive oil

¼ cup orange juice
2 tablespoons white balsamic vinegar
2 tablespoons maple syrup
2 garlic cloves, minced
1 teaspoon salt
¼ teaspoon pepper
2 green onions, finely chopped
6 ounces baby spinach
1 (15-ounce) can mandarin oranges, drained
¾ cup dried cranberries

Preparing the Quinoa
Place both kinds of quinoa in a bowl and cover with cold water. Soak for 5 minutes. Strain quinoa through a mesh strainer and rinse with cold running water.

In a medium saucepan, bring 4 cups water and quinoa to a boil over high heat. Decrease heat, cover pot and simmer until water is absorbed, about 15 minutes.

Remove from heat, fluff with fork and transfer to a serving bowl.

Preparing the Dressing
In a medium bowl, whisk together olive oil, orange juice, vinegar, maple syrup, garlic, salt and pepper. Pour over quinoa and stir until incorporated.

Putting It Together
Add green onions, spinach, mandarin oranges, and dried cranberries. Toss to coat and serve immediately.

Each serving contains 227 calories, 9g total fat, 1g saturated fat, 0g trans fat, 0mg cholesterol, 526mg sodium, 34g carbohydrate, 3g fiber, 12g sugars, 5g protein.

> Soaking and rinsing quinoa is important. The seeds are coated with saponins, which are a naturally occurring plant chemical that can cause a bitter taste. Some brands are pre-rinsed and need no further rinsing. If your package says "already rinsed," omit that step.
>
> If you prefer, quinoa can also be cooked like pasta in a large pot of boiling salted water until it blossoms. Then drain it in a fine mesh strainer.

Lime Jicama Coleslaw
Serves 4
(RECIPE BY MARY CAPONE)

A lime-mayo sauce enhances fresh, crunchy vegetables in this refreshing salad.

Ingredients
¼ cup gluten-free mayonnaise*
1 teaspoon lime juice
1 teaspoon cider vinegar
1 teaspoon maple syrup
½ red cabbage head, sliced thinly
1 small carrot, grated
¼ cup fresh jicama, grated
2 tablespoons grated white onion
Salt and pepper, to taste

Combining the Liquids
In a medium bowl, combine mayonnaise, lime juice, vinegar and syrup.

Finishing Up
Add sliced and grated vegetables to sauce and mix thoroughly. Add salt and pepper, to taste.

Cover and refrigerate at least 1 hour to chill and meld flavors before serving.

Each serving contains 105 calories, 5g total fat, 1g saturated fat, 0g trans fat, 4mg cholesterol, 142mg sodium, 15g carbohydrate, 3g fiber, 2g protein.

> *Vegenaise, a gluten-free, dairy-free, egg-free mayonnaise, is available from Follow Your Heart (followyourheart.com). For more gluten-free, allergy-friendly products, see Shopping List, page 189.

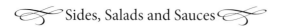
Squash and Cranberry Sage Stuffing
Serves 24
(RECIPE BY BETH HILLSON)

Bursting with flavor, this stuffing makes a nice buffet item when baked in a casserole dish. Play around with the ingredients if you wish. It works well with cornbread, pork sausage, pumpkin or whatever suits your fancy. This recipe makes enough to stuff a 10- to 16-pound bird.

Ingredients
8 cups gluten-free bread, crusts trimmed, cubed, or 8-inch-square gluten-free cornbread, cubed
3 cups diced butternut squash
3 tablespoons olive oil
3 stalks celery, chopped
4 large shallots, chopped
3 cloves garlic, minced
1½ cups fresh cranberries, washed, drained and halved
4 cooked chicken-apple sausages,* chopped (about 1 pound)
1-2 tablespoons chopped fresh sage leaves
4 teaspoons poultry seasoning
2 cups gluten-free, dairy-free chicken broth
Salt and pepper, to taste

Getting Started
Preheat oven to 300°F. Spread bread cubes over 2 cookie sheets. Toast bread in preheated oven 15 to 20 minutes or until dry, stirring occasionally. Let cool and transfer to a large mixing bowl.

Steaming the Squash
Place squash in a pan or microwave-safe dish with 1 inch of water and steam or microwave until fork tender. Drain and set aside.

Sautéing
In a large skillet, heat olive oil. Add celery, shallots and garlic and cook until vegetables soften, about 5 minutes. Add butternut squash and sauté another minute. Add cranberries and sausage and sauté until cranberries begin to soften, about 3 minutes. Add seasonings and stir.

Putting It Together
Add mixture to bread cubes and toss until well mixed. (Stuffing can be made to this point 1 day ahead and refrigerated.)

Add chicken broth and stir well. Taste and adjust seasoning, adding salt and pepper to taste.

Finishing Up
Spoon stuffing into a greased 9x13-inch baking dish. Cover baking dish with foil and bake stuffing in preheated 325°F oven for 20 minutes. Remove foil and stir stuffing. Bake 25 minutes longer or until heated through and lightly browned on top. Alternatively, use part of this recipe to stuff the cavity of a large roasting chicken or a 10- to 16-pound turkey and follow baking instructions on the poultry package. Bake any leftover stuffing as above.

Each ½ cup serving contains 151 calories, 4g total fat, 1g saturated fat, 0g trans fat, 14mg cholesterol, 158mg sodium, 25g carbohydrate, 2g fiber, 4g protein.

*If using uncooked sausage, pierce with a fork and simmer links in water for 10 minutes or until cooked through. Cool, chop and add to stuffing mixture.

Black Rice Salad
Serves 4
(RECIPE BY MATTHEW KADEY)

Antioxidant-rich Chinese black rice (also called Forbidden Rice) makes a stunning addition to mealtime. This salad works equally well for dinner or weekday lunches at the office. Try using edamame instead of lima beans, if soy is tolerated.

Ingredients
1 cup black rice
1¾ cups water
1 cup frozen lima beans
1 large carrot, sliced into matchsticks
1 cup thinly sliced radish
2 green onions, green and white parts, thinly sliced
2 sheets nori, crumbled
1½ tablespoons rice vinegar
1½ tablespoons sesame oil
Juice of ½ lemon
2 teaspoons honey
2 teaspoons wasabi powder
1 teaspoon finely minced fresh ginger
¼ teaspoon salt
2 tablespoons sesame seeds
1 avocado, thinly sliced

Getting Started
In a medium saucepan, combine rice with 1¾ cups water. Bring to a boil. Reduce heat and simmer, covered, for 30 minutes or until tender. Set aside for 5 minutes and then fluff with a fork and let cool. Meanwhile, prepare lima beans according to package directions. Drain and let cool.

Putting It Together
In a large bowl, toss together rice, beans, carrot, radish, green onion and nori.

Making the Dressing
In a small bowl, whisk together rice vinegar, sesame oil, lemon juice, honey, wasabi, ginger, and salt. Pour dressing over rice mixture and toss to coat.

Finishing Up
In a dry skillet over medium heat, toast sesame seeds until golden brown, about 3 minutes, stirring often. Divide rice salad among serving plates and top with sesame seeds and avocado slices.

Each serving contains 416 calories, 16g total fat, 2g saturated fat, 0g trans fat, 0mg cholesterol, 206mg sodium, 32g carbohydrate, 8g fiber, 6g sugars, 6g protein.

> Add the avocado just before serving to prevent it from turning brown.
>
> Nori and wasabi powder can be found in the Asian section of many supermarkets.

Capone's Marinara Sauce with Potato and Italian Sausage Gnocchi
Serves 6
(RECIPE BY MARY CAPONE)

For the flavor of fresh tomatoes, use whole canned tomatoes, not diced or puréed.

Marinara Ingredients
Makes 6 cups
2 (28-ounce) cans whole tomatoes with basil
2 tablespoons chopped fresh basil
1 tablespoon chopped fresh oregano
1 tablespoon sugar
¼ teaspoon salt, more to taste
Fresh ground pepper, to taste
¼ cup olive oil
2 cloves garlic, minced

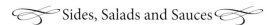

Preparing the Tomatoes

Run tomatoes through a food mill to remove skin and seeds or push by hand through a colander into a 6-quart saucepan. Discard tomato pulp left in the food mill or colander.

Making the Tomato Sauce

Warm tomatoes over medium heat and add basil, oregano, sugar, salt and pepper. Bring to a slow simmer until bubbles appear. Then cook about 20 minutes, stirring frequently, until tomato sauce resembles a thin oatmeal. Do not overcook.

Finishing Up

Taste and adjust seasoning accordingly. Add more herbs for additional flavor, if desired. If sauce is too sweet, add a pinch of salt and pepper. If it's too salty, add a pinch of sugar.

In a small pan, heat oil and add minced garlic. Cook until lightly brown or just beginning to color. Stir oil and garlic into sauce.

Each ½ cup serving contains 67 calories, 5g total fat, 1g saturated fat, 0g trans fat, 0mg cholesterol, 236mg sodium, 7g carbohydrate, 1g fiber, 1g protein.

Potato and Italian Sausage Gnocchi

Serves 6

Don't be put off by homemade gnocchi. This delicious dish is quite easy to make. For a vegetarian option, omit the sausage. This recipe can be made egg-free.*

1½ pounds baking potatoes (about 4 medium)
1 cup Mary's All-Purpose Flour Blend
(page xiv)
½ teaspoon xanthan gum
1 egg*

¾ teaspoon salt
¼ teaspoon ground nutmeg, optional
½ pound gluten-free Italian-style sausage,
casing removed, cooked and diced

Making the Potatoes

In a large pot, boil potatoes with skin on until they are easily pierced with a fork. Drain and peel.

Put potatoes through a food mill or grate them on the large side of a cheese grater onto a clean work surface.

Making the Dough

Combine flour blend and xanthan gum. Add to potatoes and knead dough, forming a mound with a well in the center, like the shape of a bird's nest.

Break egg in the center and add salt, nutmeg and sausage. Knead dough until ingredients are well incorporated. (Depending on what kind of potato you use, your dough may be too sticky to handle. If so, add a little more flour blend after you add the egg.) Dough should be smooth and stay together when rolling. Dust your work surface lightly with flour blend, adding only enough to handle dough.

Rolling the Dough

Divide dough into 4 parts. Roll each part into a long, sausage-like shape about 1½ inches in diameter. With a knife or pastry cutter, cut each long roll into individual dumplings, each about 1 inch long.

Forming the Gnocchi

Set fork face down on the end of your board. Gently roll each gnocchi over the back of the fork prongs.

Finishing Up
Bring a large pot of salted water to boil. Drop in a few gnocchi at a time, only enough to fill the bottom of the pot in a single layer. Gnocchi will soon rise to the surface of the water. Cook for an additional 2 to 3 minutes. Remove gnocchi with a slotted spoon to a serving platter.

To the Table
Cover with Capone's Marinara Sauce or your favorite tomato sauce. Serve immediately.

> Each serving contains 324 calories, 13g total fat, 4g saturated fat, 0g trans fat, 64mg cholesterol, 582mg sodium, 42g carbohydrate, 2g fiber, 10g protein.

> For **Egg-Free Gnocchi,** omit 1 egg. Combine 1 tablespoon arrowroot with 2 teaspoons water to create a paste. Add to dough in place of 1 egg.
>
> Pressed for time? Caesar's Pasta (caesarspasta.com) and Conte's Pasta (contespasta.com) offer prepared gnocchi that is gluten-free. For more gluten-free, allergy-friendly products, see Shopping List, page 189.

Carrots with Thyme and Marsala
Serves 6 to 8
(RECIPE BY MARY CAPONE)

Root vegetables add just the right flavor to a special meal and take only minutes to prepare.

Ingredients
2 tablespoons butter or non-dairy alternative
4 large carrots, sliced
1 teaspoon minced fresh thyme
Dash of salt
Pepper, to taste
¼ cup Marsala wine, optional

Getting Started
In a medium saucepan, melt butter.

Sautéing the Carrots
Add sliced carrots, thyme, salt and pepper and sauté until lightly colored, about 3 minutes. Add Marsala wine and sauté until wine reduces by half, about 5 minutes. Transfer to platter and serve warm.

> Each serving contains 69 calories, 4g total fat, 2g saturated fat, 0g trans fat, 10mg cholesterol, 50mg sodium, 6g carbohydrate, 1g fiber, 1g protein.

Green Bean Casserole
Serves 8 to 10
(RECIPE BY JULES SHEPARD)

With a few substitutions, you can enjoy this favorite Thanksgiving casserole every day. This dish travels well; garnish with "fried" onions just before serving.

"Fried" Onions
1 medium onion, sliced into thin rings
⅓ cup *Living Without's* All-Purpose Flour Blend (page xiv)
¼ teaspoon xanthan gum
¼ teaspoon sea salt

Casserole
1 pound green beans, canned or fresh
2 tablespoons unsalted butter or non-dairy alternative
2 large portobello mushrooms, sliced
½ teaspoon freshly ground black pepper
½ teaspoon garlic powder
¼ teaspoon ground nutmeg
2 tablespoons *Living Without's* All-Purpose Flour Blend (page xiv)
⅓ cup sour cream or non-dairy sour cream alternative
2 cups gluten-free, dairy-free cream of mushroom soup

Making the Onions
Preheat oven to 475°F. Lightly grease a baking sheet and set aside. Combine onion slices, ⅓ cup flour blend, xanthan gum and salt in a large bowl, tossing until onions are evenly coated. Pour out onto prepared baking sheet, separating onion rings. Bake in preheated oven for 15 to 20 minutes until golden brown, tossing 1 or 2 times. Remove from oven and set aside while you prepare the casserole.

Making the Casserole
To make the casserole, turn oven temperature down to 400°F.

If using fresh beans, boil them in lightly salted water for 5 minutes. Rinse with cold water and drain. If using canned beans, rinse, drain and set aside.

In a large saucepan, melt the butter. Toss in sliced mushrooms and stir over medium heat for 5 minutes.

Add spices and flour, stirring to coat. Cook an additional minute and add sour cream and soup. Reduce heat to medium-low and cook while mixture thickens, about 5 to 8 minutes more.

Finishing Up
Remove saucepan from heat and stir in half the "fried" onions and the drained beans.

Pour mixture into a large casserole dish and cook in preheated oven for 10 minutes or until bubbly. Sprinkle remaining prepared onions on top and bake an additional 5 minutes. Serve warm.

Each serving contains 120 calories, 7g total fat, 3g saturated fat, 0g trans fat, 10mg cholesterol, 383mg sodium, 13g carbohydrate, 2g fiber, 3g protein.

Pressed for time? Top this casserole with gluten-free Funyuns Onion-Flavored Rings, available from Frito-Lay (fritolay.com). For more gluten-free, allergy-friendly products, see Shopping List, page 189.

Super-Quick Chili Mac and Cheese
Serves 6
(RECIPE BY BETH HILLSON)

This recipe is designed for busy days when time is limited. To add a bit of fire, use hot sausage. For even more zip, stir in a small can of chopped green chilis.

Ingredients
3 cups (12 ounces) dried rice, corn or quinoa elbow pasta or 3-4 cups (8-10 ounces) other short pasta, uncooked
3-4 hot or mild chicken, turkey or pork sausages (about 1 pound)
1½ cups frozen corn kernels
1 cup gluten-free, dairy-free chicken broth
2½ cups shredded nacho/taco cheese or non-dairy cheese substitute, divided

Getting Started
Lightly oil a deep microwave-safe dish (7½x11-inch, 9x13-inch or 9-inch round).

Cooking the Pasta
Cook pasta in salted water for half the time specified on package. Pasta should be under-cooked (slightly opaque but not brittle). Drain and transfer to prepared baking dish.

Sautéing the Meat and Corn
While pasta is cooking, remove sausage from its casing and crumble into a well-oiled saucepan. Sauté meat until brown, breaking up pieces with the back of a spoon as sausage

cooks. Add corn, stirring to combine.

Putting It Together
Using a wooden spoon, gently fold meat mixture into pasta.

Adding the Cheese
Heat chicken broth in the saucepan until hot but not boiling. Remove from heat and add 2 cups cheese. Stir until smooth and pour over pasta. Gently toss to coat.

Finishing Up
Top mixture with remaining cheese. Cover dish with a moist paper towel and microwave on medium-high for 5 minutes or until bubbly. Cool 5 minutes before serving.

Each serving contains 431 calories, 12g total fat, 5g saturated fat, 0g trans fat, 44mg cholesterol, 683mg sodium, 64g carbohydrate, 5g fiber, 20g protein.

Mushroom Gravy
Makes 3 to 4 cups
(RECIPE BY BETH HILLSON)

With mushrooms and wine, this gravy brightens up any chicken or turkey dish. Pair with Maple Cider Vinegar Glazed Roasted Turkey on page 106. Garnish with fresh thyme, if desired.

Ingredients
Juices and pan drippings from roasted turkey or chicken, if available
3 tablespoons olive oil
2 large shallots, minced
1 large carrot, peeled and thinly sliced or shredded
2 stalks celery, chopped
6-8 large shiitake mushrooms, stems removed, caps sliced

½ teaspoon dried thyme
Salt and pepper
½ cup white wine
1½ cups gluten-free, dairy-free chicken broth
3 tablespoons cornstarch
4-5 tablespoons heavy cream or milk of choice
Fresh thyme, for garnish, optional

Getting Started
Collect juices from turkey or chicken from roasting pan. Cool and skim off fat.

Sautéing the Vegetables
In a saucepan, heat the oil and sauté shallots, carrot and celery over low heat until soft, about 3 minutes. Add mushrooms, thyme and salt and pepper, and sauté an additional 2 minutes or until mushrooms begin to soften. Add wine and simmer until reduced slightly. Add chicken broth and pan juices. Bring to a simmer and cook 2 to 3 minutes.

Thickening the Gravy
In a small bowl, combine cornstarch and heavy cream or milk of choice. Stir cornstarch mixture slowly into simmering vegetable liquid until gravy thickens. (You may not need to add all the cornstarch mixture.) Serve warm.

Each tablespoon contains 14 calories, 2g total fat, 1g saturated fat, 0g trans fat, 3mg cholesterol, 31mg sodium, 2g carbohydrate, 0g fiber, 0g protein.

Pierogi
Makes 48 pierogi
(RECIPE BY REBECCA REILLY)

When people with a Polish connection must give up gluten, one of their first requests is a replacement for pierogi. This traditional Polish version of stuffed dumplings is a favorite of many, regardless of heritage. The dumplings are made with a delicate dough that's rolled as thin as possible and filled with any number of sweet or savory ingredients. Boiled or sautéed, versatile pierogi can be stuffed with traditional fillings like potato and cheese (here), sauerkraut or mushrooms, or filled with cinnamon and cheese and served for dessert. This recipe can be made egg-free.*

Ingredients
3 cups *Living Without's* High-Protein Flour
Blend, more for sprinkling (page xiv)
¼ teaspoon salt
⅛ teaspoon xanthan gum
3 large eggs*
1 tablespoon oil of choice
¾ cup hot water
Potato, Cheese and Onion Filling

Making the Dough
In a large bowl, mix together flour blend, salt and xanthan gum. Make a well in the center.

Crack eggs into the well and add oil. Using a fork, mix eggs and oil together. Slowly mix in hot water, being careful not to "cook" the eggs. As you're mixing, incorporate dry ingredients.

Use your hands to gather the dough into a ball. Dough should be soft but not sticky. Chill dough if not using immediately.

Rolling the Dough
Place 2 sheets of heavy-duty plastic wrap (or an extra-large zip-top plastic bag cut into 2 pieces) on a flat surface. Sprinkle flour blend on plastic wrap and place dough in the center. Sprinkle more blend over dough and place another sheet of plastic wrap on top. Roll out dough to ⅛-inch thickness.

Forming the Pierogi
Cut circles of dough (2 inches for small pierogi, 3 to 3½ inches for large pierogi) with a round cookie cutter or drinking glass. Place a teaspoon of Potato, Cheese and Onion Filling on each round. Fold the dough over, forming a semi-circle. Press edges together with the tines of a fork.

Finishing Up
Place pierogi, a few at a time, in a large pot of boiling water. Cook for 6 minutes. Remove pierogi with a slotted spoon and drain.

Saute in butter or oil or enjoy as is.

> For **Egg-Free Pierogi,** omit 3 eggs. Mix 2 tablespoons flax meal with 6 tablespoons warm water; let sit 5 minutes until slightly thickened. Add this mixture to ¾ cup hot water in the recipe and continue as instructed. Add 1 to 2 additional tablespoons of water if dough is too dry to mix.
>
> Store uncooked pierogi in the refrigerator for several days or freeze up to 3 months.

Potato, Cheese and Onion Filling
Makes 4 cups
This filling works well with peeled red potatoes. For added taste, stir in chopped fresh parsley and crisp bacon bits.

Ingredients
1½ pounds potatoes, scrubbed and peeled
1-2 large onions, finely chopped
2 tablespoons butter or oil
8 ounces grated sharp cheddar cheese or non-dairy alternative, optional
Salt and fresh pepper

Boiling the Potatoes
Bring a large pot of salted water to a boil. Add
potatoes and cook until tender but still firm,
about 15 minutes. Drain and mash.

Sautéing
While potatoes are boiling, sauté onion in
butter or oil in a small skillet until soft and
translucent.

Finishing Up
Mix mashed potatoes with sautéed onions. Add
cheddar cheese, if used. Taste and adjust salt
and pepper, as desired. Cool and fill pierogi.

Each pierogi contains 68 calories, 3g total fat, 1g saturated
fat, 0g trans fat, 19mg cholesterol, 47mg sodium, 9g
carbohydrate, 0g fiber, 2g protein.

Desserts
Cakes and Pies

"The secret to staying satisfied on a gluten-free or allergy-friendly
diet is to demand more, not less, of your food."

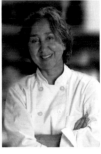

Recipes by
Mary Capone
and other celebrity chefs

Mary Capone

Boulder, Colorado

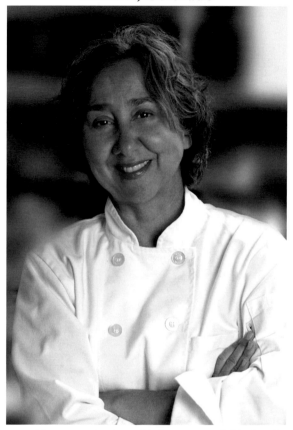

"I like to spend hours creating in my kitchen surrounded by loved ones and laughter, filling long tables with delicious platters of food."

I spent hours in the kitchen when I was a child. Before I could even reach the stove, I sat on a stool and stirred bubbling pots of sauce with my dad. I fried *centi fritti* (Italian cookies) with my Aunt Carmel. I baked elegant angel food cakes with beatific buttercreams with my Aunt Lillian. It was in the kitchens of my Italian relatives that I learned that food was an expression of love. I was hooked on the delicious treats of my heritage.

As a young adult, I started Marie's Crepes, a European-style kiosk that offered Parisian-style crepes. That's when my health began to falter. I eventually discovered I had celiac disease and had to remove all gluten from my diet. I felt better immediately but I wondered how I could indulge my passion for baking and eating exquisite food when I had to give up gluten. Wonderful cakes and desserts felt like part of my genetic makeup—my birthright!

I began a journey to discover just how many delicious foods I could reshape and recreate. I worked with gluten-free flour blends until I created one that satisfied my pastry flour standards. Soon I developed a sixth sense about what would work for my desserts and what would fail, a confidence that allowed me to fearlessly create dishes more enticing than the original recipes.

I became a bully in my kitchen, pushing ingredients to their highest potential and shaping foods in new ways. I chose bright ingredients to create deep dimensions of flavor. I started with wholesome ingredients, stone-ground flours, seasonal vegetables and fruits and fresh herbs and spices. I used the highest quality extracts and oils.

When it comes to food, I admit that I am a hedonist. I crave rich, savory dishes with bold flavors, salty comfort foods and decadent and beautifully textured desserts. I discovered that the secret to staying satisfied on a gluten-free or allergy-friendly diet is to demand more—not less—of your food.

Whether you're a seasoned gluten-free baker or just starting out, don't be afraid to roll up your sleeves and dive into creating scrumptious desserts. Gluten-free, allergy-friendly recipes can rise far above the foods you ate before. They can remind you to enjoy the sensual pleasures of the table. You deserve it.

Mary Capone is a gluten-free baking expert, cooking teacher and business owner. In 2005, she launched The Wheat Free Gourmet Cooking School, where she teaches gourmet gluten-free cooking and baking. In 2010, she founded Bella Gluten-Free, a company that produces allergy-free baking mixes that contain gluten-free whole grain flours.

Capone is the author of *The Gluten-Free Italian Cookbook* (The Wheat Free Gourmet Press).

Where to find Mary Capone:
bellaglutenfree.com

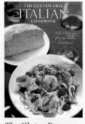

The Gluten Free Italian Cookbook is available at LivingWithout.com.

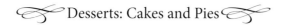

Cakes and Pies

Mary's
Royal Banana Cake with Mocha Frosting
Serves 16

A favorite for birthday gatherings, this banana cake is very easy to make. The balance of rich mocha frosting and moist, slightly sweet cake is a flavor combination that everyone will love. The chocolate chips are a delightful addition to the batter. Decorate the top with more. This recipe can be made egg-free.*

Ingredients
3 cups Mary's All-Purpose Flour Blend (page xiv)
1 teaspoon xanthan gum
1½ teaspoons sea salt
1½ teaspoons baking powder
½ teaspoon baking soda
1 cup granulated sugar
1 cup lightly packed brown sugar
1 cup vegetable oil, such as grapeseed or canola
3 large eggs,* room temperature
1 tablespoon pure vanilla extract
2 cups mashed ripe bananas**
1 cup coconut milk or plain yogurt or non-dairy yogurt alternative
1½ cups chocolate chips

Getting Started
Preheat oven to 350°F. Grease two 9-inch round cake pans and line with parchment paper.

Making the Batter
In a large bowl, whisk together Mary's Baking Blend, xanthan gum, salt, baking powder and baking soda. Set aside.

In the bowl of a heavy-duty stand mixer, blend sugars and oil together until combined. Add eggs one at a time just until incorporated. Add vanilla and blend.

Add dry ingredients a little at a time, stopping mixer to scrape sides of

*For **Egg-Free Royal Banana Cake,** omit 3 eggs. Add 2 tablespoons arrowroot powder to the dry ingredients. Combine 1 tablespoon flax meal with 3 tablespoons warm water. Let sit for 5 minutes until slightly thickened and then add to the rest of the wet ingredients. Note: If using 1 cup coconut milk (not yogurt), use ¼ cup coconut milk instead of 3 tablespoons warm water to make the flax meal mixture. Add remaining ¾ cup coconut milk to the bananas later in recipe, as instructed.

**To ripen bananas quickly, microwave one banana at a time for 30 seconds until it feels soft.

For sugar that's less refined and with a lower glycemic index, try organic coconut palm sugar or organic evaporated cane juice.

bowl down when needed. Add bananas and coconut milk or yogurt and mix to blend. Do not over-mix. Gently fold in chocolate chips.

To the Oven and Out
Distribute batter evenly between 2 prepared cake pans. Smooth top of batter with a knife.

Place pans in preheated oven and bake for 35 minutes or until center is set. Let cool in cake pans for 10 minutes. Invert pans onto a cooling rack and peel off parchment paper. Cool completely before frosting.

Gluten-free, allergy-friendly chocolate chips are available from Enjoy LIfe Foods (enjoylife-foods.com). For other gluten-free, allergy-friendly ingredients, turn to Shopping List, page 189.

Mocha Buttercream Frosting
Enough frosting for two 9-inch cakes

8 tablespoons (1 stick) unsalted butter or dairy-free alternative, room temperature
2½–3 cups confectioners' sugar, more to reach desired thickness
1 teaspoon pure vanilla extract
2 tablespoons brewed espresso coffee* or extra-strong coffee
2 tablespoons unsweetened cocoa powder
¼ teaspoon salt
Chocolate chips or chocolate candies, for decoration

*A single shot of espresso at your local coffee shop is equivalent to 2 tablespoons.

Making the Frosting
With a mixer, beat butter and sugar together until smooth. Add vanilla, coffee, cocoa powder and salt. Beat until blended.

Assembling the Cake
Place first cake layer on a cake stand and add 1¼ cups frosting to top. Spread evenly to sides. Add second layer and top with remaining frosting. Cover top and sides completely. Sprinkle top with chocolate chips or chocolate candies of your choice.

Each serving contains 605 calories, 29g total fat, 11g saturated fat, 0g trans fat, 55mg cholesterol, 353mg sodium, 86g carbohydrate, 3g fiber, 48g sugars, 4g protein.

Mary's
Blueberry Lemon Cake with Crumble Crust
Serves 12 to 16

This recipe combines the bright flavors of blueberries and lemon to create a beautiful spring cake that is as simple to make as it is good to eat. The crumble topping, laced with vibrant lemon zest, becomes the bottom crust. It's sure to be a hit at your next gathering. This cake can be made egg-free.*

Ingredients

⅓ cup brown sugar
2½ cups fresh blueberries or fresh berries of choice
1 tablespoon lemon juice
1 cup coconut milk or milk of choice
1½ cups vegetable oil, such as grapeseed or canola
1½ cups granulated sugar, such as organic evaporated cane juice
3 large eggs,* room temperature
2 teaspoons lemon extract
1 teaspoon pure vanilla extract
2¼ cups Mary's All-Purpose Flour Blend (page xiv)
2 teaspoons baking powder
1 teaspoon xanthan gum
½ teaspoon sea salt
½ teaspoon baking soda
Confectioners' sugar, for dusting cake

Crumble

1¼ cups Mary's All-Purpose Flour Blend (page xiv)
¾ cup granulated sugar, white or light brown
2 teaspoons lemon zest
¼ teaspoon salt
5 tablespoons butter or non-dairy alternative, room temperature, cut into small pieces

Getting Started
Preheat oven to 350°F. Spray a 9-inch springform pan and line with parchment paper.

Distributing the Berries
Evenly distribute ⅓ cup of brown sugar onto lined springform pan. Place berries evenly on top of the sugar. Set pan aside.

*For **Egg-Free Blueberry Lemon Cake,** omit 3 eggs. Add 2 tablespoons arrowroot to dry ingredients. Combine 1 tablespoon flax meal with 3 tablespoons warm water or warm coconut milk. Let sit for 5 minutes until slightly thickened before adding to the rest of the wet ingredients.

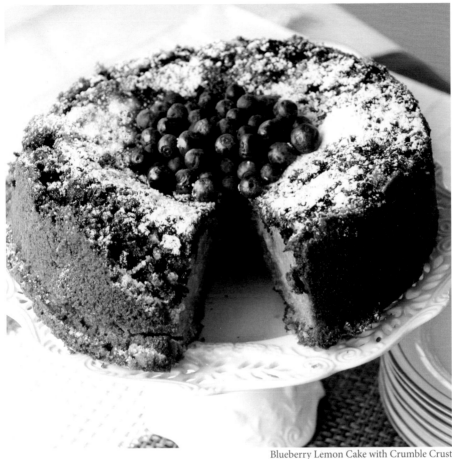

Blueberry Lemon Cake with Crumble Crust

Making the Milk Mixture
Add lemon juice to coconut milk in a small bowl. Let sit for 5 minutes until it becomes lumpy. (Some fat-free milks will not form lumps.)

Blending the Egg Mixture
With a heavy-duty stand mixer, blend oil and sugar together until combined. Add eggs one at a time just until incorporated. Add extracts and blend.

Putting It Together
In a medium bowl, whisk together Mary's Baking Blend, baking powder, xanthan gum, salt and baking soda. Add milk mixture and flour mixtures to batter, alternating. Stir until batter is smooth. Do not over-mix. Pour batter into prepared pan.

Making the Crumble Topping
In a medium bowl, whisk together flour blend, sugar, lemon zest and

Some fat-free milk will not thicken when lemon juice is added. The acid from the lemon still helps tenderize the cake, producing a delicate crumb.

salt. Cut in butter with a pastry cutter or rub in with fingers until streusel begins to clump together. Sprinkle crumble evenly over top of prepared batter.

To the Oven and Out
Place in preheated oven and bake for 1 hour and 20 minutes or until center is set. Let cool for 10 minutes. Invert pan onto a cake plate and peel off parchment paper.

Dust generously with confectioners' sugar while still warm. Let cool before cutting.

The vibrant lemon crumble topping becomes the crust when it is baked and inverted.

Each serving contains 564 calories, 33g total fat, 10g saturated fat, 0g trans fat, 63mg cholesterol, 216mg sodium, 65g carbohydrate, 1g fiber, 35g sugars, 3g protein.

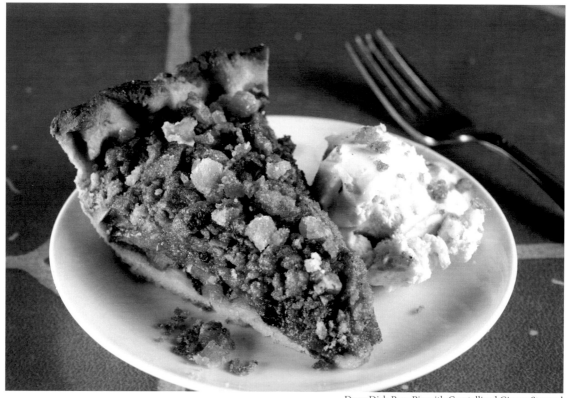

Deep Dish Pear Pie with Crystallized Ginger Streusel

Mary's
Deep Dish Pear Pie with Crystallized Ginger Streusel
Serves 8 to 10

Fresh pears are one of my favorite dessert ingredients. Baked, poached, in a cobbler and of course, in pear pie, the fragrant and slightly sweet taste is always a winner. The ginger streusel makes for a beautiful presentation and adds a lovely spicy note to the pie. This Pastry Crust can be made egg-free.*

Pastry Crust
Makes one 9-inch pie crust

1 cup Mary's All-Purpose Flour Blend (page xiv)
2 tablespoons sweet rice flour or tapioca starch/flour
3 tablespoons granulated sugar
¼ teaspoon salt
6 tablespoons unsalted butter or non-dairy
alternative, well chilled
1 large egg*
1 tablespoon water, more as needed

Getting Started
Lightly grease a 9-inch glass pie plate. Set aside.

Making the Dough
In a food processor, mix flour blend, sweet rice flour, sugar and salt. Pulse to blend.

Add butter and pulse just until mixture resembles coarse meal.

Add egg and water, and mix just until dough forms a ball.

Flatten dough into a 6-inch disk and place between 2 sheets of dusted parchment or waxed paper. Refrigerate for 30 minutes. While dough is chilling, prepare Pear Filling and Streusel Topping (next page).

Finishing Up
Preheat oven to 375°F. Remove the dough from the refrigerator and roll it out between parchment paper into an 11-inch round. Place dough in prepared pie plate and crimp the border. Add the Pear Filling. Spread Streusel Topping evenly over Pear Filling.

Use this pastry crust recipe for all your pie creations.

*For **Egg-Free Pastry Crust,** omit 1 egg. Combine 1 tablespoon flax meal with 3 tablespoons warm water. Let sit for 5 minutes until slightly thickened before adding to the rest of the ingredients. Dust hands with gluten-free flour when handling dough.

Why use a glass pie plate?
Glass heats more slowly and evenly than metal. If you use a metal pie pan, check the pie a few minutes before it finishes baking as the crust may brown more quickly.

To the Oven and Out

Place pie in preheated oven and bake for 35 to 40 minutes or until pears are cooked and streusel is a golden brown. If top becomes too brown, cover loosely with foil. Serve warm with ice cream, if desired.

Pear Filling

¼ cup pure maple syrup or ginger syrup
½ cup water
½ cup dark brown sugar
½ teaspoon sea salt
4-5 pears, such as Bosc or Anjou, peeled and sliced
2 teaspoons potato starch (not potato flour)
¼ cup currants, optional
1 teaspoon ground cinnamon
2 tablespoons fresh lemon juice

Making the Pear Filling

In a medium saucepan, simmer syrup, water, brown sugar and salt until mixture thickens slightly, about 3 minutes. In a medium bowl, toss pears in potato starch and coat well.

Add pears, currants, cinnamon and lemon juice to syrup mixture. Simmer until fruit is coated with a thickened syrup and is partially cooked, about 5 minutes. Remove from stove and let cool slightly. Add to prepared pie crust.

Streusel Topping

¾ cup Mary's All-Purpose Flour Blend (page xiv)
½ cup brown sugar
¼ cup crystallized ginger,* minced, or ½ teaspoon ground ginger
½ teaspoon ground cinnamon
¼ teaspoon ground cardamom
4 tablespoons butter or non-dairy alternative, room temperature,
cut in pieces

*Crystallized ginger and ginger syrup can be found at most health food stores or online at gingerpeople.com.

Making the Streusel Topping

In a small bowl, mix together flour blend, brown sugar, ginger, cinnamon and cardamom. Cut in butter with a pastry cutter until mixture is crumbly.

Each serving contains 416 calories, 14g total fat, 8g saturated fat, 0g trans fat, 55mg cholesterol, 195mg sodium, 74g carbohydrate, 4g fiber, 42g sugars, 2g protein.

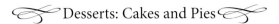

Mary's
Parisian Puff Pastry
Makes 12 pastries

I dream of my visits to Paris, sitting in a steamy café filled with the rich aromas of coffee and bittersweet chocolate. The smell of butter was so dense, it seemed to drip from the air. Inspired by the buttery-crisp shell of French pastries, I worked hard to create this gluten-free light, puff pastry dough. It can be formed into envelope-style pastries or rolled into Danish-style pastries. Once you get the hang of it, add your own fillings. So put on a beret, make a cup of café au lait, and eat pastry to your heart's content. This recipe can be made egg-free.*

Ingredients
1 cup Mary's All-Purpose Flour Blend (page xiv), more for dusting
½ teaspoon xanthan gum
½ teaspoon sea salt
1 cup water
6 tablespoons (¾ stick) unsalted butter or non-dairy alternative
3 tablespoons sugar
Pinch of freshly grated nutmeg
4 large eggs*
1 large egg white beaten with 1 teaspoon water, optional
3 tablespoons confectioners' sugar, for dusting, optional

Getting Started
Line 2 baking sheets with parchment paper or lightly grease them.

Combining the Dry Ingredients
Blend flour blend, xanthan gum and salt. Set aside.

Making the Butter Mixture
In a medium saucepan, heat water, butter, sugar and nutmeg over medium heat until butter is melted.

Combining the Mixtures
Immediately add dry ingredients to butter mixture and stir until dough forms. Cook for 2 minutes over low heat, stirring constantly. Pour mixture into the bowl of a food processor fitted with a steel blade and let cool slightly.

*For **Egg-Free Parisian Puff Pastry,** omit 4 eggs. Combine 4 tablespoons flax meal with 9 tablespoons warm water. Let sit until cool. Add 2 teaspoons baking powder to flax meal mixture, stirring 3 to 4 times to combine. Let the dough in the food processor cool slightly. Then add the flax meal mixture and pulse until smooth. Note: This dough will be sticky. For easier handling and rolling out, dust extra gluten-free flour on the dough and on your hands. Bake egg-free pastries until edges are golden brown.

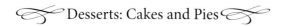

Add eggs, and pulse until incorporated. The dough should be smooth and elastic.

Working the Dough
Place dough on a piece of parchment paper that's been lightly dusted with gluten-free flour. Lightly dust the top of the dough ball with additional flour. Place a piece of parchment paper over dough and roll it out into a 9x16-inch rectangle or about ¼-inch thick throughout. Chill in the refrigerator for 30 minutes for easier handling.

Finishing Up
Preheat oven to 325°F. Remove top parchment paper and cut dough into 3x4-inch rectangles. Add about 1 tablespoon of desired filling and fold dough in 2 corners, crimping it together in the middle.

Dust fingers with gluten-free flour if you need to handle dough. Brush with egg wash, if desired. Place pastries on prepared baking sheets.

To the Oven and Out
Place in preheated oven and bake for 20 to 25 minutes or until pastries are golden brown on the outside. Turn off the oven and let dry for an additional 30 minutes. This allows the inside of the pastries to dry and hollow. Remove from oven and sprinkle pastries with confectioners' sugar, if desired.

Each serving contains 141 calories, 8g total fat, 4g saturated fat, 0g trans fat, 86mg cholesterol, 123mg sodium, 16g carbohydrate, 0g fiber, 5g sugars, 3g protein.

Filling Variations
Cheese Danish: Mix ¾ cup of cream cheese or dairy-free alternative with 1 tablespoon confectioners' sugar. Add 1 tablespoon of cream cheese mixture and 1 teaspoon of fresh fruit or your favorite jam to pastry dough rectangles.

Fold dough into an envelope shape and pinch to seal.

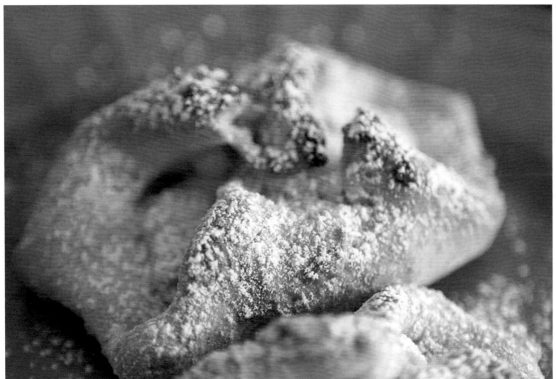

Parisian Puff Pastry

Pain Au Chocolat: Add 1 tablespoon of chocolate chips to each rectangle of pastry dough.

Fold dough into an envelope shape and pinch to seal.

Pain Aux Raisin: Do not cut the rolled-out dough into rectangles. Spread ½ cup of gluten-free almond paste on top of rolled-out dough and sprinkle with ½ cup raisins that have been soaked in about ¼ cup cognac or brandy for several hours or overnight. With long side facing you, roll the dough into a log and cut into 12 pieces. Separate and turn onto cut side. Brush with egg wash, if desired, and bake as recipe instructs.

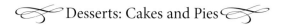

Nonna's Dark Chocolate Cake
Serves 24
(RECIPE BY MARY CAPONE)

The moist, rich center of this festive cake complements the crusty chocolate outside. Sprinkle confectioners' sugar on top and place fresh raspberries, strawberries or candied fruit around the rim. Cut cake into thin slices and it will serve a crowd. Recipe can be halved for a smaller group. For best results, do not replace the eggs in this recipe.

Ingredients
12 ounces bittersweet chocolate
1¾ cups (3½ sticks) unsalted butter or non-dairy alternative
12 large eggs, separated
2 cups sugar
2 teaspoons pure vanilla extract
1½ teaspoons gluten-free raspberry extract
¼ cup Mary's All-Purpose Flour Blend (page xiv)
1 teaspoon xanthan gum
½ cup unsweetened cocoa powder
½ teaspoon salt
Confectioners' sugar, for dusting

Getting Started
Preheat oven to 325°F. Lightly grease a 10-inch springform pan. (Use an 8½ or 9-inch pan if recipe is halved.)

Melting Chocolate and Butter
In a double boiler, melt chocolate. Remove from heat and let cool about 10 minutes.

In a small saucepan, melt butter. Remove from heat and let cool about 10 minutes.

Making the Egg Mixture
Separate eggs. Place whites into a large bowl and set aside. Place yolks into the large bowl of a mixer and beat them until they turn light yellow, about 1 minute. Add sugar and beat until mixture drops from a spatula in a heavy ribbon, about 5 to 7 minutes.

Add vanilla and raspberry extracts to yolks and mix on slow speed just until ingredients are incorporated.

Adding the Chocolate
Fold in melted chocolate and butter with a large spoon or rubber spatula just until mixed.

Making the Flour Mixture
In another bowl, whisk together dry ingredients. Sprinkle on top of batter and fold in gently.

Whipping the Egg Whites and Combining
Whip egg whites to soft peaks and fold into batter just until whites are mixed. Pour batter into prepared pan.

To the Oven and Out
Bake in preheated oven for 75 minutes. If using the half recipe, bake for 50 minutes. Cake will rise like a soufflé and fall when it cools. Let it cool completely and then sprinkle with confectioners' sugar and decorate with fruit of choice.

Each serving contains 301 calories, 24g total fat, 14g saturated fat, 0g trans fat, 141mg cholesterol, 138mg sodium, 24g carbohydrate, 3g fiber, 6g protein.

A traditional soufflé is served piping hot directly from the oven. This cake, however, is better after it sits and literally collapses, creating an uneven crusty top and a soft, delicate center. To achieve this, just let cake cool.

Strawberry Crostata
Makes one 8-inch crostata
(RECIPE BY MARY CAPONE)

A simple fruit crostata is the perfect way to end a special meal. What's not to love about sweet shortbread pastry dough wrapped around fresh fruit? Use strawberries or a fruit of your choice. This Sweet Pastry Crust can be made egg-free.*

Filling
2 cups fresh or frozen strawberries, hulled and sliced
3 tablespoons sugar
1 tablespoon potato starch (not potato flour)
1 teaspoon lemon zest

Sweet Pastry Crust
1 cup Mary's All-Purpose Flour Blend (page xiv)
2 tablespoons tapioca starch/flour
3 tablespoons sugar
¼ teaspoon salt
6 tablespoons unsalted butter or non-dairy alternative, well chilled
1 large egg*
1 tablespoon ice water, more as needed

Getting Started
In a small bowl, mix together berries, sugar, potato starch and zest. Set aside.

Making the Crust
To make the crust, in a food processor or large bowl, mix together flour, tapioca starch, sugar and salt. Cut in butter just until mixture resembles a coarse meal. Add egg and ice water and mix until dough forms a ball. Place dough between 2 pieces of parchment paper and flatten dough to about a 4-inch disk. Refrigerate for 30 minutes.

Preheat oven to 350°F. Lightly grease a 9-inch pie pan.

Preparing the Crust
Roll out dough between 2 sheets of parchment paper to form a 9- to 10-inch circle. Peel off top sheet. Transfer crust to prepared pie pan, dough side down. Peel off remaining sheet of parchment.

Adding the Strawberry Filling
Place strawberry mixture on crust and gently fold pastry up and over the edge of the filling, pleating it as you go. You will end up with about an 8-inch crostata.

To the Oven and Out
Place pan in preheated oven and bake for 30 to 35 minutes until crust is a golden brown. Cool before serving.

Each serving contains 207 calories, 9g total fat, 6g saturated fat, 0g trans fat, 49mg cholesterol, 11mg sodium, 29g carbohydrate, 1g fiber, 2g protein.

*For **Egg-Free Sweet Pastry Crust**, omit 1 egg. Combine 1 tablespoon flax meal with 3 tablespoons warm water. Let sit for 5 minutes until slightly thickened before adding to the ice water and mixing the dough.

Peppermint Brownie Pie
Makes one 9-inch pie
(RECIPE BY ROBERT LANDOLPHI)

The best of both worlds in every bite, this delightful combination of chocolate and mint makes a unique holiday pie. The crust can be made several days ahead; the finished pie can be made the day before serving. For best results, do not replace the eggs in the filling.

Basic Pie Crust
1¾ cups *Living Without's* High-Protein Flour Blend (page xiv)
1 tablespoon sugar

1½ teaspoons xanthan gum
½ teaspoon baking soda
½ teaspoon salt
¼ cup vegetable shortening
3 tablespoons cold butter or non-dairy alternative
3 tablespoons coconut milk or milk of choice

Filling
¾ cup butter or dairy-free alternative
4 ounces unsweetened (baking) chocolate
2 cups sugar
3 large eggs
¾ teaspoon mint extract
1 cup *Living Without's* High-Protein Flour Blend (page xiv)

Getting Started
Grease a 9-inch pie pan.

In a medium bowl, whisk together flour, sugar, xanthan gum, baking soda and salt. Add shortening and butter to the flour mixture. Using your fingertips, a pastry blender or 2 butter knives, rub or cut the shortening and butter into the dry ingredients until mixture is the texture of coarse meal with pea-size pieces. Gradually stir in the milk with a fork to moisten the dry ingredients.

Forming the Dough
On a lightly floured cutting board, form the dough into a ball, wrap with plastic wrap and refrigerate for at least 1 hour or up to a week.

Preparing the Pie Crust
Place the dough between 2 pieces of waxed paper and roll into a 12-inch round. Remove the waxed paper from the top of the round and invert the prepared pie plate on top of the dough. Place your other hand under the waxed paper and turn the round over so that the dough falls into the pan. Tuck the dough into the pan and peel off the waxed paper. Let the overhang drape over the edge of the pie plate, while gently fitting the dough into the pan.

Using scissors, trim the dough to a 1-inch overhang. Fold the overhang under evenly. Crimp the edges of the pie crust with your thumb and forefinger or press it with the tines of a fork.

Refrigerate the crust until ready to fill.

Making the Filling
Preheat oven to 350°F.

In a large microwaveable bowl, microwave butter and chocolate on high for 2 minutes. Stir with a wooden spoon and then microwave for 30 more seconds. Stir until chocolate is completely melted and smooth.

Mix in sugar, eggs and mint extract. Gradually stir in flour until blended.

To the Oven and Out
Pour batter evenly into unbaked pie crust. Place in preheated oven and bake for 55 to 60 minutes or until a toothpick inserted in the center comes out clean.

Remove from oven and allow pie to cool completely before cutting and serving.

Each serving contains 573 calories, 33g total fat, 18g saturated fat, 1g trans fat, 112mg cholesterol, 207mg sodium, 71g carbohydrate, 2g fiber, 5g protein.

Apple Custard Crumb Pie
Serves 8
(RECIPE BY BETH HILLSON)

This recipe's creamy custard center offers a unique and luscious twist on traditional apple pie. Replacing the sour ceam with a dairy-free substitute works well. Prepare Flaky Pie Crust before making the filling and topping or use a prepared gluten-free pie crust, if desired. This recipe can be made egg-free.*

Streusel Topping
½ cup packed light brown sugar
¾ cup *Living Without's* All-Purpose Flour Blend (page xiv)
½ teaspoon ground cinnamon
¼ teaspoon salt
6 tablespoons cold unsalted butter or non-dairy alternative, cut into small pieces

Filling
5 McIntosh apples
⅔ cup low-fat sour cream, non-dairy alternative or coconut yogurt
1 large egg,* lightly beaten, or 3 additional tablespoons sour cream + 1 tablespoon cornstarch or potato starch
½–¾ cup sugar, to taste
3 tablespoons *Living Without's* All-Purpose Flour Blend (page xiv) or rice flour
1 teaspoon ground cinnamon
¼ teaspoon salt
1 Flaky Pie Crust, unbaked

Making the Streusel Topping
To make Streusel Topping, combine all topping ingredients in a food processor and pulse until mixture resembles coarse meal. Reserve.

Getting Started
Preheat oven to 350°F. Peel and thinly slice apples.

Making the Egg Mixture
In a large mixing bowl, combine sour cream and egg (or egg replacement) and beat well.

Combining the Dry Ingredients
In another bowl, combine sugar, flour, cinnamon and salt. Whisk into sour cream mixture. Add apple slices, tossing to coat.

Putting It Together
Spread mixture over unbaked Flaky Pie Crust. Sprinkle Streusel Topping over the top.

To the Oven and Out
Set the pie on a cookie sheet for ease of handling. Place on middle rack in preheated oven and bake 55 to 60 minutes or until filling is bubbly and topping is brown. If crust browns too quickly, cover edges loosely with foil.

Each serving contains 555 calories, 26g total fat, 13g saturated fat, 0g trans fat, 134mg cholesterol, 436mg sodium, 80g carbohydrate, 3g fiber, 4g protein.

Flaky Pie Crust
Makes one 9-inch crust
1½ cups + 2 tablespoons *Living Without's* High Protein Flour Blend (page xiv)
1 tablespoon potato flour (not potato starch)
1 teaspoon xanthan gum
¼ teaspoon salt
2-3 teaspoons sugar
½ teaspoon baking powder
½ teaspoon ground cinnamon
4 tablespoons butter or non-dairy alternative
4 tablespoons organic shortening
1 large egg* or 2 tablespoons additional unsweetened applesauce
1 teaspoon cider vinegar
2 tablespoons unsweetened applesauce

Getting Started

In the bowl of a food processor fitted with the knife blade, pulse dry ingredients to combine. Cut butter and shortening into pieces. Sprinkle over dry ingredients. Pulse several times until pieces are the size of large peas.

Making the Dough

In a separate bowl, combine egg, vinegar and applesauce. Add to flour mixture and blend just to combine. Carefully gather dough into a ball. (Watch your fingers as steel knife is very sharp.) Wrap in plastic wrap and chill at least 1 hour.

Finishing Up the Crust

Place the dough between 2 layers of plastic wrap and press it down with heel of hand. Starting from the middle, roll dough out uniformly in all directions to form a 9-inch circle. Rotate the dough in quarter turns to help even-out the dough to about ¼-inch thickness throughout.

Carefully peel off the top layer of plastic wrap. Turn the crust into the pan, slowly peeling off the backing. Crimp the edges to create a finished look.

Each serving contains 190 calories, 13g total fat, 6g saturated fat, 0g trans fat, 26mg cholesterol, 175mg sodium, 17g carbohydrate, 1g fiber, 2g protein.

> Unless rolled too thin, this dough is not prone to tearing. If it does, pull it back into place and pat it down.

Apple Spice Cake
Serves 16
(RECIPE BY DIANE KITTLE)

This cake is a good reason to head to the orchards for apples. Filled with shredded apples and spices, it will last several days refrigerated. To forego frosting, bake it in a large bundt pan

(75 minutes in 350°F preheated oven) and top with a dusting of confectioners' sugar. This recipe can be made egg-free.*

Ingredients
5 large eggs,* room temperature
1½ cups canola oil or vegetable oil
2 cups sugar or organic evaporated cane juice
3½ cups Dee's Pastry Flour Blend (page xiii)
2 teaspoons baking soda
1 teaspoon baking powder
1 tablespoon ground cinnamon
1 teaspoon ground nutmeg
1 teaspoon salt
1 teaspoon xanthan gum
3 cups grated apples

Getting Started

Preheat oven to 350°F. Grease two 8- or 9-inch round cake pans and dust with gluten-free flour.

Making the Egg Mixture

In the bowl of an electric mixer, beat eggs, oil and sugar at medium-high speed for 3 minutes. Mixture will thicken and appear pale yellow.

Making the Flour Mixture

On a piece of waxed paper, sift together the flour, baking soda, baking powder, cinnamon, nutmeg, salt and xanthan gum.

Combining Mixtures and Apples

Add the dry ingredients to the wet batter and mix on medium-low speed just until blended, about 30 seconds. Squeeze grated apples in between paper towels to remove some of the juice and add apples to mixture. Blend just until smooth.

To the Oven and Out

Divide the batter evenly between the 2 prepared

pans. Place in preheated oven and bake for about 1 hour to 1 hour and 15 minutes. (Time will vary depending on oven and pan size.) Cake is done when an inserted toothpick comes out clean. Let cake cool in the pan for 20 minutes. Then turn it out of the pans to cool completely before frosting.

Frosting the Cake

Cake layers will be 2-plus inches high. Frost as a 2-layer cake or cut each cake horizontally into 2 layers for a 4-layer cake. Frost the cake with either Vanilla Buttercream Frosting or Spiced Buttercream Frosting.

Each slice as a bundt cake without frosting contains 439 calories, 23g total fat, 2g saturated fat, 0g trans fat, 66mg cholesterol, 353mg sodium, 56g carbohydrate, 2g fiber, 4g protein.

*For **Egg-Free Apple Spice Cake**, omit 5 eggs. Combine 5 tablespoons flax meal with 15 tablespoons of warm water. Let sit for 5 minutes until slightly thickened. Then add to the rest of the wet ingredients.

Vanilla Buttercream Frosting
Makes 8½ to 9 cups

This frosting is not too sweet. The "buttercream" will fill most of a 5-quart mixing bowl.

6 cups confectioners' sugar or organic powdered evaporated cane juice
½ teaspoon salt
½ cup boiling water
2½ cups vegetable shortening
12 tablespoons (1½ sticks) butter or non-dairy alternative, cut into 1-inch pieces
1 tablespoon pure vanilla extract

Making the Frosting

In the bowl of an electric mixer, fitted with whisk attachment, combine sugar and salt.

Add boiling water and beat at low speed until smooth and cool, about 5 minutes.

Add shortening and butter to the sugar mixture and beat at medium speed until smooth, about 3 minutes. Increase speed to medium-high and beat until light, fluffy and increased in volume, about 10 minutes.

Each serving (2 tablespoons) contains 120 calories, 9g total fat, 4g saturated fat, 0g trans fat, 4mg cholesterol, 36mg sodium, 10g carbohydrate, 0g fiber, 0g protein.

*For **Spiced Buttercream Frosting**, place 6 cups Vanilla Buttercream Frosting in a bowl. Add 1 teaspoon each ground cinnamon and ground nutmeg. Blend well by hand.

Carrot Cake
Serves 12
(RECIPE BY DIANE KITTLE)

Simple to make, this carrot cake looks and tastes special but you don't need a special occasion to whip it up. It pairs well with Spiced Buttercream Frosting (above). This recipe can be made egg-free.*

Ingredients
Gluten-free flour, for dusting
4 large eggs,* room temperature
¾ cup canola oil or vegetable oil
2 cups sugar or organic evaporated cane juice
2½ cups Dee's Pastry Flour Blend (page xiii)
1 tablespoon baking powder
1 teaspoon baking soda
2 teaspoons ground cinnamon
1 teaspoon salt
1 teaspoon xanthan gum
2 cups grated carrots
1 (14-ounce) can crushed pineapple, drained with ½ cup juice reserved
6 cups Spiced Buttercream Frosting

Getting Started

Preheat oven to 350°F. Grease two 7- or 8-inch round cake pans and dust with gluten-free flour.

Making the Egg Mixture

In the bowl of an electric mixer, beat the eggs, oil and sugar at medium-high speed for 3 minutes. Mixture will thicken and look pale yellow.

Making the Flour Mixture

On a piece of waxed paper, sift together the flour blend, baking powder, baking soda, cinnamon, salt and xanthan gum.

Combining Mixtures, Carrots and Pineapple

Add the dry ingredients to the egg mixture and mix on medium-low speed just until blended, about 30 seconds. Add grated carrots, pineapple and reserved pineapple juice. Mix until blended, another 30 seconds. Scrape sides of the bowl well with a rubber spatula and blend by hand until all ingredients are incorporated.

To the Oven and Out

Divide the batter evenly between 2 prepared pans. Place pans in preheated oven and bake about 50 minutes to 1 hour. (Time will vary depending on oven and pan size.) Cake is done when an inserted toothpick comes out clean. Let cake cool in the pan for 20 minutes. Then turn cake out of pans to cool completely before frosting with Spiced Buttercream Frosting (page 161).

Each slice without frosting contains 421 calories, 16g total fat, 2g saturated fat, 0g trans fat, 70mg cholesterol, 454mg sodium, 67g carbohydrate, 2g fiber, 4g protein.

*For **Egg-Free Carrot Cake,** omit 4 eggs. Combine 4 tablespoons flax meal with 12 tablespoons warm water. Let sit for 5 minutes until slightly thickened. Then add to the rest of the wet ingredients.

Chocolate Raspberry Torte
Serves 18
(RECIPE BY DIANE KITTLE)

With berries in the batter, in the filling and on top, this torte packs a triple raspberry punch. It's the perfect dessert for a special celebration or to impress guests at your next dinner party. Tortes are traditionally served in very thin wedges. Slice the torte down the middle; then cut into 1- to 2-inch wedges. This recipe can be made egg-free.*

Ingredients
Gluten-free flour, for dusting
2½ cups fresh raspberries or 1 (14-ounce) bag frozen raspberries, thawed
1 cup rice milk or milk of choice, very warm
1 tablespoon cider vinegar
3 cups Dee's Pastry Flour Blend (page xiii)
1 cup unsweetened cocoa powder
1 tablespoon + 1 teaspoon baking soda
1 teaspoon salt
1 teaspoon xanthan gum
2 large eggs*
⅔ cup canola oil or vegetable oil
2 cups sugar or organic evaporated cane juice
2 teaspoons pure vanilla extract
1 (12-ounce) jar seedless raspberry jam, fruit sweetened, divided
7 cups Vanilla Buttercream Frosting, divided (page 161)
1 cup fresh raspberries, for filling and decoration
Grated chocolate, optional

Getting Started

Preheat oven to 350°F. Grease two 9-inch round cake pans and dust with gluten-free flour.

Making the Raspberry Purée

Place 2½ cups fresh or thawed raspberries in a food processor or blender and process until smooth. Strain mixture through a fine mesh sieve into a small bowl, discarding seeds. You should have 1 cup of purée. Set aside.

Making the Milk Mixture
Combine warm milk and vinegar in a small bowl. Set aside.

Making the Flour Mixture
On a piece of waxed paper, sift together flour blend, cocoa powder, baking soda, salt and xanthan gum. Set aside.

Making the Egg Mixture
In the bowl of an electric mixer, beat eggs, oil and sugar at medium-high speed for 3 minutes.

Finishing Up
Add milk mixture, raspberry purée and vanilla extract to egg mixture and mix for 1 minute. Add sifted dry ingredients to wet ingredients in mixer and blend on low speed just to mix. Then increase speed to medium and mix for 2 minutes. Scrape down sides of bowl and mix for an additional 30 seconds.

Spoon batter equally into prepared cake pans.

To the Oven and Out
Place pans in preheated oven and bake for 40 to 55 minutes. Cake is done when an inserted toothpick comes out clean. (Time will vary depending on oven and pan size). Remove from oven and cool cake in pans for 20 minutes. Then turn cakes out of the pans onto a wire rack to cool completely before frosting.

Assembling the Torte
To assemble and decorate the torte, cut each layer with a knife horizontally to create a total of 4 layers. Place the bottom layer on a flat cake plate or on a 9-inch cardboard circle. Spoon half the jam onto the layer, spreading evenly to cover.

Place 1 cup Vanilla Buttercream Frosting in a small bowl and add 8 to 10 raspberries to make raspberry frosting. Blend together with a spoon until berries break up and are mixed into the frosting.

Place the next cake layer on the torte. Spoon all the raspberry frosting onto this layer, spreading evenly over the surface. (Alternatively, reserve some frosting for decoration.) Add the next layer of cake and spread the remaining jam over it. Place the final cake layer on the torte, top side up.

Finishing Up
Frost torte with remaining 6 cups of Vanilla Buttercream Frosting. To finish, pipe a border of reserved raspberry frosting around the base of the torte, if desired. Then pipe rosettes around the top of the torte, placing a fresh raspberry on top of each rosette. For a final touch, sprinkle shaved chocolate lightly over the top of the torte, if desired.

Each slice without frosting contains 288 calories, 10g total fat, 1g saturated fat, 0g trans fat, 23mg cholesterol, 418mg sodium, 49g carbohydrate, 4g fiber, 3g protein.

Each slice with frosting and jam contains 694 calories, 38g total fat, 13g saturated fat, 0g trans fat, 36mg cholesterol, 531mg sodium, 89g carbohydrate, 4g fiber, 3g protein.

*For **Egg-Free Chocolate Raspberry Torte**, omit 2 eggs. Combine 2 tablespoons flax meal with 6 tablespoons warm water. Let sit for 5 minutes until slightly thickened before adding to oil and sugar.

Cranberry Mousse Pie
Makes one 9-inch pie
(RECIPE BY BETH HILLSON)

If you want a refreshing way to enjoy cranberries, this not-too-sweet dessert is just the thing. It's as festive as it is delicious. Decorate with whipped cream or non-dairy whipped topping. Garnish with chocolate shavings and cranberries.

Ingredients
½ pound fresh or frozen cranberries
½ cup sugar, divided
¼ cup orange juice
1½ teaspoons dried orange peel
¼ teaspoon ground ginger
2 tablespoons Triple Sec, other orange liqueur
or additional orange juice
½ tablespoon unflavored gelatin, softened in
1 tablespoon orange juice
1 cup whipping cream or non-dairy
whipped topping*
1 Chocolate Graham Cracker Crust

Getting Started
In a medium saucepan, combine cranberries, ¼ cup sugar, orange juice, orange peel and ground ginger. Bring to a boil, stirring frequently.

Lower heat to medium-low and cook, stirring frequently until cranberries break down, about 15 minutes. Remove from heat.

Add Triple Sec and stir. Let cool slightly.

Making the Gelatin Mixture
Warm gelatin and orange juice mixture in the microwave for 10 seconds or until it liquefies. Pour into the cranberry mixture in a steady stream, stirring while adding. Scrape into a bowl and chill about 20 minutes.

Finishing Up
With an electric mixer, beat cream and remaining ¼ cup sugar until stiff. Fold into cranberry mixture and spoon into Chocolate Graham Cracker Crust. Chill at least 3 hours before serving.

*If using sweetened non-dairy whipped topping, omit ¼ cup sugar.

Chocolate Graham Cracker Crust
Makes one 9-inch crust

This easy crust goes with any sweet pudding or mousse-textured filling. It can be made several days ahead and stored in the refrigerator until ready to use.

1 cup gluten-free graham cracker crumbs
1 tablespoon unsweetened cocoa powder
¼ cup sugar
3 tablespoons melted butter or
non-dairy alternative
½ cup chocolate chips
2 tablespoons light cream or
coconut milk

Getting Started
Preheat oven to 325°F. Lightly grease the bottom of an 8- or 9-inch springform pan or a tart pan with removable bottom.

Making the Graham Cracker Crust
Combine graham cracker crumbs, cocoa and sugar in a medium bowl. Add melted butter and stir until crumbs are moistened. Press mixture into the bottom of prepared pan.

Place pan on the middle rack in preheated oven and bake 12 minutes for a 9-inch pan, 15 minutes for an 8-inch pan. Remove from oven and cool.

Finishing Up

In a microwave-safe bowl, combine chocolate chips and cream. Heat on medium for 1 minute or until chips are softened. Blend together until smooth. Spread mixture over cooled crust. Chill until set before adding Cranberry Mousse Filling.

Serves 8. Each serving contains 272 calories, 16g total fat, 10g saturated fat, 0g trans fat, 36mg cholesterol, 26mg sodium, 35g carbohydrate, 2g fiber, 22g sugars, 2g protein.

White Cupcakes
Makes 28 to 30 cupcakes
(RECIPE BY JULES SHEPARD)

These cupcakes are light and airy. Easily doubled, this recipe can be baked in advance and frozen. Work in batches to make as many cupcakes as you need to match your guest list. Estimate high, as guests are going to sneak seconds. This recipe can be made egg-free.*

3 cups *Living Without's* All-Purpose Flour Blend (page xiv)
¼ cup dry milk powder or non-dairy milk powder alternative
1 tablespoon baking powder
¼ teaspoon salt
½ cup butter or non-dairy alternative
2 cups sugar
4 large eggs*
2 teaspoons pure vanilla extract
1 cup milk or non-dairy milk of choice (vanilla flavor preferred)

Getting Started

Preheat oven to 350°F. Line 28 to 30 muffin tins with decorative cupcake papers.

Making the Flour Mixture

In a large bowl, whisk together flour blend, milk powder, baking powder and salt and set aside.

Preparing the Batter

In a large mixing bowl, combine the butter and sugar, beating well with the paddle attachment until the mixture is very light and fluffy (about 3 to 4 minutes). Add the eggs 1 at a time, beating well after each addition. Mix in the vanilla with the last egg addition. Slowly add the milk, alternating with the flour mixture and beating in between the additions. Beat batter until smooth.

To the Oven and Out

Pour batter into prepared muffin tins. Place in preheated oven and bake for about 20 minutes. Cupcakes are done when a toothpick inserted into the middle comes out clean and cupcakes begin to pull away slightly from the sides of the pans. When done, turn off the oven and leave the oven door open to let the cupcakes slowly cool there for 10 minutes or so. Then remove them to a cooling rack.

Frosting the Cupcakes

When fully cooled, frost the cupcakes with Bourbon Buttercream Frosting or frosting of choice. Alternatively, wrap cupcakes in waxed paper or plastic wrap and seal inside freezer bags to freeze until ready to use.

Bourbon Buttercream Frosting
Makes 4 cups

Bourbon adds an unexpected tang to this rich frosting, making ordinary icing worthy of any special occasion. This frosting sets up nicely once applied. For best results, top cupcakes when frosting is prepared, as it becomes stiff and crunchy if left to sit in the bowl.

1 cup butter or non-dairy alternative, slightly softened

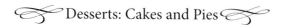

4 cups confectioners' sugar
⅓ cup milk or non-dairy milk of choice (vanilla flavor preferred)
¼-⅓ cup bourbon
1 tablespoon pure vanilla extract

Making the Frosting

Beat butter at medium speed with an electric mixer until creamy. Gradually add confectioners' sugar, alternating with milk, ¼ cup bourbon and vanilla, beating on low speed until incorporated after each addition. If the frosting is too stiff, whip in the remaining bourbon (up to total ⅓ cup). If the frosting is too thin, beat in ½ cup additional confectioners' sugar.

Each cupcake without frosting contains 148 calories, 4g total fat, 2g saturated fat, 0g trans fat, 37mg cholesterol, 84mg sodium, 27g carbohydrate, 0g fiber, 2g protein

Each cupcake with frosting contains 273 calories, 10g total fat, 6g saturated fat, 0g trans fat, 54mg cholesterol, 86mg sodium, 43g carbohydrate, 0g fiber, 2g protein.

*For **Egg-Free Cupcakes,** omit 4 large eggs. Add 4 tablespoons arrowroot powder to dry ingredients. Add 4 tablespoons unsweetened applesauce to beaten butter and sugar mixture. Proceed with recipe instructions.

For **Chocolate Cupcakes,** add ¼ cup unsweetened cocoa powder to dry ingredients; replace 1 cup vanilla-flavored milk with 1¼ cups chocolate milk of choice.

Desserts
Bars, Cookies and More

"Creating a dessert that suits a friend's or family member's
special diet is a form of love."

Recipes by
Rebecca Reilly
and other celebrity chefs

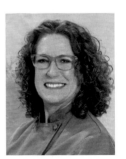

Rebecca Reilly

Watertown, Massachusetts

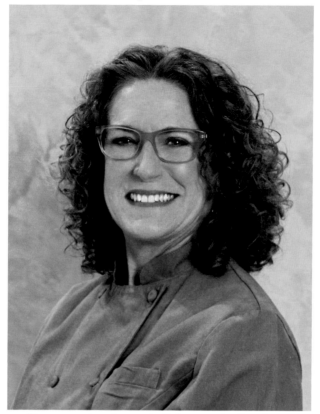

"Progress, not perfect...and a little sweet rice flour."

My gluten-free journey began in 1991 when my son Reilly was born. He had trouble settling down and did not nurse well. I was forced to stop nursing early and substituted soy formula. For the next five years, Reilly suffered from chronic ear infections, strep throat, congestion, a swollen belly, low weight and more. His pediatrician kept prescribing antibiotics and discounted my question, "Could this child have food allergies?"

Eventually, I turned to alternative medicine and ended up putting Reilly on an elimination diet with a rotational menu. For a month, I joined him at school for lunch so he would have company eating his "weird" food. His friends thought it was cool that his mom was having lunch

PHOTO BY LEXI COPITHORNE

with him. When he began to flourish on a diet that avoided gluten and other items, I knew I had made the right decision.

A year later, my daughter and I were tested for food allergies. Our issues were not as complicated as Reilly's but gluten was on our avoid list. That's when our home became completely gluten free. I began translating all my family recipes and my mother joined me in developing gluten-free pasta and preparing gluten-free meals for all of us. I saw that creating foods that suit someone's special diet was a form of love. My son thrived, my daughter's headaches lessened and I found a new culinary direction.

At first, I couldn't even pronounce some of the ingredients in gluten-free baking, let alone understand their function. Much of this type of baking was counterintuitive to my classical gluten-filled culinary training. But I kept experimenting and taking notes. I tried new flours and noted how they behaved. Once I incorporated one ingredient I liked, I found I was using it over and over in other recipes. Finally, I achieved success in recreating favorite desserts without gluten and dairy.

Rebecca Reilly graduated from Le Cordon Bleu Culinary School and from master classes at Le Nôtre Pâtissier in Paris. She ran The Madd Apple, a popular restaurant and café in Portland, Maine, and Rebecca's Kitchen, a catering firm. Reilly now offers private catering and teaches gluten-free baking classes at the Natural Gourmet Institute in New York City.

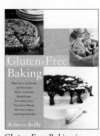

Reilly is author of *Gluten Free Baking: More Than 125 Recipes for Delectable Sweet and Savory Baked Goods, Including Cakes, Pies, Quick Breads, Muffins, Cookies, and Other Delights* (Simon & Schuster).

Gluten Free Baking is available at LivingWithout.com.

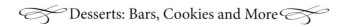

Bars, Cookies and More

Rebecca's
Grilled Brandied Peach Shortcakes
Serves 6

A lively marriage of flavors makes this comfort food one you will never forget.

Shortcakes
Makes 6 biscuits

1½ cups *Living Without's* All-Purpose Flour Blend (page xiv),
more to knead dough
2 tablespoons sugar
1 tablespoon baking powder
3½ teaspoons spice blend*
½ teaspoon xanthan gum
¼ teaspoon salt
6 tablespoons cold unsalted butter or non-dairy alternative,
cut into pieces
¾-1 cup milk of choice, more for brushing tops
2 teaspoons ground cinnamon
2 tablespoons sugar

Getting Started
Preheat oven to 425°F. Line a baking sheet with parchment or a Silpat.

Making the Dough
Mix together flour blend, sugar, baking powder, spice blend, xanthan gum and salt in a bowl.

Cut the butter into the flour mixture with a pastry cutter or your fingertips until the largest pieces are the size of peas.

Make a well in the center of the flour and pour the milk into the well. Mix with a fork until the dough is evenly moistened and just combined. It should still feel a little dry but not too crumbly.

Working the Dough
Gently knead by hand 5 or 6 times to create a loose ball.

*Spice Blend
3 tablespoons ground cinnamon
1 teaspoon allspice
1 teaspoon ground ginger
¼ teaspoon ground cloves
Mix all the spices together and store in a tightly covered container.

A Silpat is a reusable silicone-coated sheet developed by French pastry chefs. It creates an instant, no-stick surface for rollling out pastry dough and for baking.

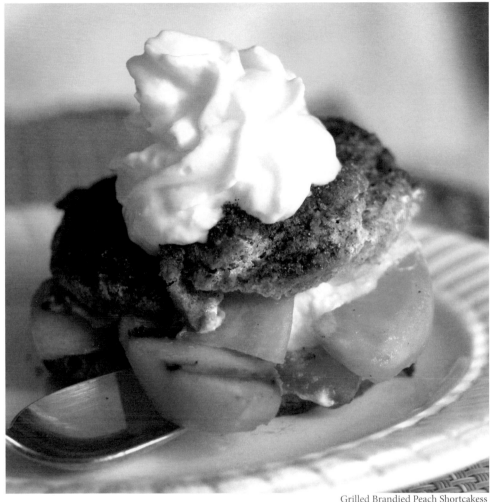
Grilled Brandied Peach Shortcakess

Turn the dough out onto a lightly floured work surface and pat it into a square. Use a floured 3-inch biscuit cutter to cut the dough into 6 biscuits.

Baking the Shortcake
Transfer the biscuits to prepared baking sheet leaving 2 inches between each biscuit.

Brush tops with milk. Combine 2 teaspoons cinnamon and 2 tablespoons sugar and sprinkle over the tops.

Place in preheated oven and bake 18 to 20 minutes until the biscuits are golden brown. Cool on a cooling rack, while preparing peaches.

Serve brandied peaches with shortcake biscuits or enjoy them alone with a dollop of non-dairy ice cream or whipped cream.

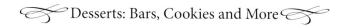

Grilled Brandied Peaches

Serves 6

2½ ounces brandy
1 tablespoon butter or non-dairy alternative, melted
1 tablespoon honey
3 firm ripe peaches, pitted and halved
Whipped topping of choice

Getting Started
Combine the brandy, butter and honey.

Grilling the Peaches
Place peach halves, cut side down, on grill rack coated with cooking spray. Grill 2 minutes on each side or until grill marks appear.

Remove peaches from grill; thinly slice and place in a bowl. Stir in the brandy-honey mixture.

Assembling the Shortcakes
Just before serving, split the biscuits in half and evenly spoon the peaches over the bottom half of each biscuit.

Place biscuit tops over the peaches. Crown the top of each biscuit with a dollop of whipped topping and serve.

Each serving contains 88 calories, 2g total fat, 1g saturated fat, 0g trans fat, 5mg cholesterol, 0mg sodium, 12g carbohydrate, 1g fiber, 10g sugars, 1g protein.

Shortcake Biscuits and Brandied Peaches can be made a day ahead. Store biscuits in a zip-top plastic bag on the counter and refrigerate peaches in their sauce. Assemble just before serving.

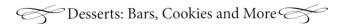

Rebecca's
Coconut Oatmeal Cookies
Make 36 cookies

These cookies are delicious by themselves or they can be filled with Chocolate Ganache (page 174) for mouthwatering cookie "sandwiches." They freeze well unfilled. This recipe can be made egg-free.*

Ingredients
3 cups gluten-free old-fashioned oats, uncooked
1 cup *Living Without's* All-Purpose Flour Blend (page xiv)
½ teaspoon xanthan gum
¾ teaspoon salt
½ teaspoon baking powder
½ teaspoon baking soda
1 cup unsweetened flaked coconut
¾ cup vegetable shortening
¾ cup brown sugar or coconut sugar
¾ cup sugar
1 large egg*
1 teaspoon pure vanilla extract
¼ cup coconut water or water

Getting Started
Preheat oven to 350°F. Lightly grease cookie sheets.

Mixing the Ingredients
Mix together oats, flour blend, xanthan gum, salt, baking powder, baking soda and coconut.

In a separate bowl, beat together shortening and sugars until light and fluffy. Beat in egg, vanilla and coconut water.

Stir dry ingredients into creamed mixture.

To the Oven and Out
Drop batter by rounded teaspoons onto prepared cookie sheets. Place in preheated oven and bake 12 to 15 minutes.

Let cookies cool 5 minutes before removing from cookie sheet.

*To make **Egg-Free Coconut Oatmeal Cookies,** omit 1 egg. Mix 1 tablespoon flax meal with 3 tablespoons hot water; let sit 5 minutes until thickened. Add to recipe to replace 1 egg.

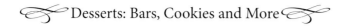

Chocolate Ganache Filling
Makes 1 cup

½ cup unsweetened canned coconut milk
6 ounces dark chocolate, chopped
2 tablespoons cold unsalted butter or cold non-dairy alternative
4 tablespoons confectioners' sugar, more as needed

Getting Started
In a small, heavy saucepan, heat coconut milk just until it starts to simmer.

Making the Filling
Take the pan off the heat and add chocolate, shaking pan gently to immerse the chocolate into the hot coconut milk. Add cold butter. Let mixture stand for 1 minute. Then beat with a wire whisk until chocolate and butter dissolve and mixture is smooth. Refrigerate until mixture is cold.

Whip again with a wire whisk until fluffy. Add confectioners' sugar, as needed, until mixture is of frosting consistency.

Assembling the Cookie Sandwiches
To assemble cookies, spread some filling onto a cookie. Press another cookie on top of filling. Continue until all cookies are filled and paired. Let cookies sit before serving to allow the ganache to set. For a firmer filling, refrigerate frosted cookies.

Each cookie without filling contains 151 calories, 9g total fat, 4g saturated fat, 0g trans fat, 6mg cholesterol, 157mg sodium, 17g carbohydrate, 1g fiber, 1g protein

Each cookie with ganache filling contains 324 calories, 18g total fat, 8g saturated fat, 1g trans fat, 17mg cholesterol, 175mg sodium, 39g carbohydrate, 2g fiber, 3g protein.

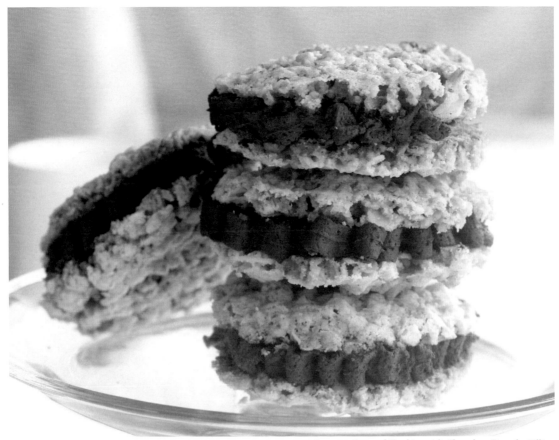

Coconut Oatmeal Cookies with Chocolate Ganache Filling

Rebecca's
Chocolate Mint Bars
Makes 36 cookies

This recipe may seem long but actual preparation is very easy—and well worth it. These cookies can be made egg-free.* They freeze well.

Crust
1 cup *Living Without's* All-Purpose Flour Blend (page xiv)
⅛ teaspoon salt
¼ teaspoon xanthan gum
½ cup (1 stick) unsalted butter or non-dairy alternative
⅔ cup sugar
2 large eggs*
2 ounces unsweetened chocolate, melted
½ teaspoon pure vanilla extract

Icing
¼ cup (½ stick) unsalted butter, softened, or
non-dairy alternative
2 cups confectioners' sugar, sifted
½-1 teaspoon mint extract
3-6 tablespoons cream or milk of choice

Glaze
2 ounces bittersweet or semi-sweet chocolate
2 tablespoons unsalted butter or non-dairy alternative

Getting Started
Preheat oven to 350°F. Lightly grease a 9-inch square pan.

Making the Crust
To make crust, mix together flour blend, salt and xanthan gum.

In a separate bowl, cream butter and sugar until fluffy and white, about 5 minutes. Add eggs one at a time. Slowly mix in melted chocolate and vanilla.

Add dry ingredients to creamed mixture, mixing until just blended.

*For **Egg-Free Chocolate Mint Bars,** omit 2 eggs. Combine 2 tablespoons flax meal with 6 tablespoons hot water; let sit 5 minutes until thickened. Add to recipe to replace 2 eggs.

Don't like mint? Replace mint with orange extract.

To prevent chocolate from seizing (or thickening), melt it gently over hot (not boiling) water or melt it in the microwave on medium power for 30- to 40-second intervals.

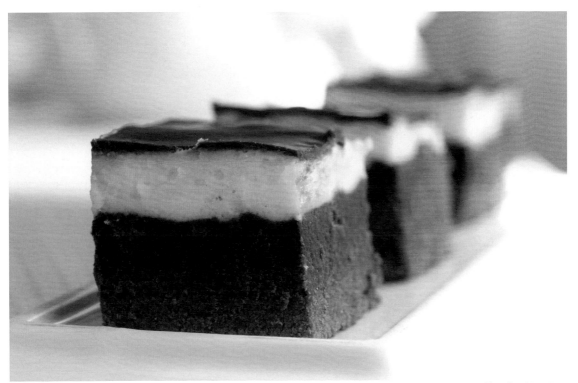

Chocolate Mint Bars

Into the Oven and Out
Pour batter into prepared pan, spreading evenly. Place in preheated oven on middle rack and bake 15 minutes or until done. Cool in the pan.

Making the Icing
To make icing, cream ¼ cup butter and confectioners' sugar. Add mint extract and enough cream to make icing a spreadable consistency.

Spread icing over cooled crust.

Making the Glaze
To make glaze, melt 2 ounces chocolate over simmering water. Remove from heat and whisk in butter until thoroughly combined.

Gently spread glaze evenly over icing. Allow glaze to harden before cutting. Cut one way across the pan in 1-inch wide slices. Then cut 4 times across in the other direction, making 36 bars.

Each cookie contains 148 calories, 9g total fat, 6g saturated fat, 0g trans fat, 34mg cholesterol,19mg sodium, 17g carbohydrate, 1g fiber, 1g protein.

Allergy-friendly chocolate is available from Enjoy Life Foods (enjoylifefoods.com). For more gluten-free or allergy-friendly products, see Shopping List, page 189.

Rebecca's
Congo Bars
Makes up to 36 bars

Congo Bars have a rich butterscotch taste. If you can eat nuts, fold some in along with the chocolate chips for a bit of added protein and crunch. These bars freeze well. This recipe can be made egg-free.*

Ingredients
2½ cups *Living Without's* All-Purpose Flour Blend (page xiv)
2 teaspoons baking powder
¼ teaspoon xanthan gum
⅛ teaspoon salt
¾ cup unsalted butter or non-dairy alternative, melted
2⅓ cups packed light brown sugar
3 large eggs*
1½ teaspoons pure vanilla extract
2 cups chocolate chips
½ cup walnuts, lightly toasted, optional

Getting Started
Preheat oven to 350°F. Lightly grease and flour a 10x10-inch or 10x15-inch pan. (Use the square pan for thicker bars.)

Mixing the Ingredients
Mix together flour blend, baking powder, xanthan gum and salt.

In separate bowl, mix together melted butter and sugar. Add eggs one at a time, beating well after each addition. Add vanilla.

Gently mix dry ingredients into liquids. Then fold in chocolate chips and walnuts, if used.

Finishing Up
Spoon batter into prepared pan, spreading evenly. Bake in preheated oven until the top is golden brown, about 25 to 30 minutes, or until done. (These bars taste better if they're slightly under-baked.)

Transfer to wire rack and let cool. Cut into bars.

Each bar contains 173 calories, 7g total fat, 4g saturated fat, 0g trans fat, 30mg cholesterol, 59mg sodium, 27g carbohydrate, 0g fiber, 2g protein.

*For **Egg-Free Congo Bars,** omit 3 eggs. Add 1 tablespoon arrowroot to dry ingredients. Combine 2 tablespoons flax meal with 6 tablespoons warm water; let sit 5 minutes until slightly thickened. Then add to recipe to replace the 3 eggs.

Rebecca's
Coconut Plum Gratin
Serves 4

This light, slightly sweet dessert is also great reheated for breakfast. Try apricots, peaches or nectarines in place of plums. If time is short, use packaged cookies instead of making macaroons.

Ingredients
8–12 Coconut Macaroons, crumbled (about 1½ cups)
3 cups diced ripe plums
2 pieces candied ginger, finely diced, optional
1 (8-ounce) container coconut yogurt or plain yogurt of choice
1 teaspoon coconut nectar, agave nectar or sugar
1 teaspoon arrowroot

Getting Started
Preheat oven to 350°F. Line a cookie sheet with parchment paper. Lightly grease 4 oven-proof ramekins.

Preparing the Cookie Crumble
Crumble the macaroons onto prepared cookie sheet, spreading crumbs evenly over the surface. Bake in preheated oven for 15 to 20 minutes to dry out the cookies. Cool.

Putting It Together
Sprinkle cookie crumbs evenly over the bottom of prepared 4 ramekins.

Evenly divide the fruit over the top of the cookies. Lightly press the fruit into the cookies. Sprinkle the diced ginger over the top.

Finishing Up
Whisk the yogurt, nectar and arrowroot together and pour over the fruit. Pop under the broiler for 1 to 2 minutes or until the topping begins to brown. Serve warm.

Replace Coconut Macaroons with gluten-free oatmeal cookies, soft molasses-ginger cookies or snickerdoodles. No need to crisp these cookies as you do with the macaroons.

Each serving contains 224 calories, 10g total fat, 8g saturated fat, 0g trans fat, 0mg cholesterol, 78mg sodium, 34g carbohydrate, 6g fiber, 20g sugars, 2g protein.

Rebecca's
Coconut Macaroons
Makes 2 dozen

Finely shredded carrots are the secret ingredient in these soft vegan macaroons. Enjoy them alone or crumble them to make Coconut Plum Gratin.

Ingredients
1 cup canned coconut milk
2 tablespoons coconut nectar or honey
⅛ teaspoon salt
⅓ cup coconut flour
1 teaspoon pure vanilla extract
2 cups sweetened shredded coconut
1 cup finely shredded carrots
2 tablespoons chia gel (1½ teaspoons chia seed*
soaked in 1½ tablespoons hot water)

*If you don't have chia seeds, replace them with an equal amount of flax meal.

Getting Started
Preheat oven to 350°F. Coat a baking sheet with parchment paper or cooking spray.

Mixing and Cooking
Whisk together the coconut milk, coconut nectar and salt in a heavy saucepan over medium heat.

Add the flour and whisk thoroughly. Heat the mixture to a full boil and continue to boil for about 1 minute or until it has thickened.

Finishing Up
Remove from the heat and stir in the vanilla, coconut, carrots and chia gel.

Drop the mixture by teaspoonsful onto prepared baking sheet. Place in preheated oven and bake for 18 to 20 minutes or until golden brown. Cool on the baking sheet.

Each serving contains 60 calories, 4g total fat, 3g saturated fat, 0g trans fat, 0mg cholesterol, 37mg sodium, 6g carbohydrate, 2g fiber, 1g sugars, 1g protein.

Apricot Chocolate Bars
Makes 16 bars
(RECIPE BY BETH HILLSON)

These bars combine chocolate and apricots to produce a chewy, decadent dessert. If you're eating nut-free, substitute crunchy rice cereal for the pecans.

Ingredients
6 ounces dried apricots (about 1 cup firmly packed), finely chopped
¼ cup granulated sugar
¾ cup water
1 teaspoon pure vanilla extract
1⅓ cups pecans (about 4 ounces), optional
1 cup *Living Without's* All-Purpose Flour Blend (page xiv)
1 teaspoon xanthan gum
⅔ cup firmly packed light brown sugar
½ teaspoon salt
⅔ cup chocolate chips*
½ cup (1 stick) cold unsalted butter or non-dairy alternative, cut into bits
Confectioners' sugar, for dusting

Making the Filling
To make apricot filling, combine apricots, sugar and water in a 1½-quart heavy saucepan over medium-high heat. Cover and simmer for 15 minutes, stirring occasionally. Remove lid and continue to simmer, stirring and mashing apricots until excess liquid is evaporated and filling thickens. Stir in vanilla. Set filling aside.

Getting Started
Preheat oven to 350°F. Line an 8-inch square baking pan with aluminum foil, leaving a 2-to 3-inch overhang on 2 opposite ends. Spray foil with vegetable oil.

Toasting the Pecans (if using)
On a separate baking sheet, toast pecans in the preheated oven until golden brown, about 5 to 7 minutes. Let cool.

Chopping the Ingredients
In a food processor, pulse pecans, flour, xanthan gum, brown sugar and salt until mixture is coarsely chopped. Add chocolate chips and butter and pulse until mixture resembles coarse crumbs.

Putting It Together
Press half the chocolate chip mixture into the bottom of prepared pan.

Spread apricot filling evenly over chocolate chip mixture.

Crumble remaining chocolate chip mixture evenly over apricot filling, pressing down slightly.

To the Oven and Out
Bake bars in preheated oven 1 hour or until golden. Remove pan from oven and cool on baking rack. Lift out of pan by aluminum foil handles. Set on a smooth surface and cut into bars. Sprinkle with confectioners' sugar and cut into bars.

Each bar contains 265 calories, 16g total fat, 6g saturated fat, 0g trans fat, 15mg cholesterol, 77mg sodium, 33g carbohydrate, 2g fiber, 2g protein.

*Allergy-friendly chocolate chips are available from Enjoy Life Foods (enjoylifefoods.com). For other gluten-free or allergy-friendly products, see Shopping List, page 189.

Cinnamon Fritters with Orange Chipotle Syrup
Makes 20 to 24
(RECIPE BY MARY CAPONE)

Serve these crispy fritters for a special dessert or breakfast. Don't forget to pass the syrup. For best results, do not replace the eggs in this recipe.

Orange Chipotle Syrup
1½ cups dark brown sugar
1 cup water
2 large navel oranges, zested and juiced (about ½ cup juice)
2 canned chipotle peppers, minced
½ teaspoon ground cinnamon

Cinnamon Fritters
1 cup water
5 tablespoons butter or non-dairy alternative
3 tablespoons sugar
½ teaspoon ground cinnamon
Pinch of salt
1 cup Mary's All-Purpose Flour Blend (page xiv)
½ teaspoon xanthan gum
4 large eggs
1 tablespoon canned green chilis
Vegetable oil, for frying
Confectioners' sugar, for dusting

Making the Syrup
To make syrup, combine sugar, water, orange zest and juice and peppers in a medium saucepan. Bring to boil. Reduce heat to simmer until syrup thickens and coats the back of a spoon, about 15 minutes. Stir in cinnamon. Set aside.

Making the Fritter Dough
To make fritters, combine water, butter, sugar, cinnamon and salt in medium saucepan. Bring to boil.

Lower heat and add flour blend and xanthan gum, stirring with a wooden spoon until ingredients are combined and mixture pulls away from sides of pan. Remove from heat and let cool, about 5 minutes.

Beating the Fritter Dough
Add dough to a stand mixer with paddle attachment, food processor with blade or a large bowl with a hand mixer. Begin beating mixture at low speed, adding eggs one at a time. Mix until eggs are fully absorbed and dough is smooth and bounces to touch. Stir in chilis just until combined. Dough will be sticky.

Finishing Up
Pour about 2 inches of oil into a deep frying pan or wok. Heat to about 350°F.

Working in batches, drop 1 heaping teaspoon of fritter dough into hot oil. Cook, turning frequently until fritters puff to 3 times their size, about 6 minutes. Drain on a baking sheet lined with paper towels. Repeat with remaining dough.

Mound hot fritters on a serving plate and dust with confectioners' sugar. Serve with warm Orange Chipotle Syrup.

Each fritter contains 126 calories, 4g total fat, 2g saturated fat, 0g trans fat, 42mg cholesterol, 31mg sodium, 21g carbohydrate, 0g fiber, 1g protein.

Chili Pepper Brownies
Makes 20 brownies
(RECIPE BY MARY CAPONE)

These scrumptious brownies combine chili peppers and chocolate with the rich flavors of cinnamon and vanilla. For best results, do not replace the eggs in this recipe.

Ingredients
¾ cup Mary's All-Purpose Flour Blend
(page xiv)
¾ teaspoon xanthan gum
⅛ teaspoon salt
1⅓ cups sugar or evaporated cane juice
½ cup unsweetened cocoa powder
¼ teaspoon baking soda
1 teaspoon ground cinnamon
3 large eggs, room temperature
8 tablespoons unsalted butter or non-dairy
butter alternative
¾ teaspoon ground chili powder or 3-4 small
dried New Mexico chili peppers
¼ cup vegetable oil of choice
1 tablespoon pure vanilla extract
⅓ cup chocolate chips*

Getting Started
Preheat oven to 350°F. Lightly grease a 9x9-inch pan and line with parchment paper.

Mixing It Together
In a medium bowl, whisk together dry ingredients. Add eggs, one at a time and blend with a wooden spoon or hand mixer.

In a small saucepan, melt butter. Add chili powder or whole dried chili peppers. Simmer for 3 to 5 minutes to infuse chili flavor into butter. If using whole chilis, remove them from butter after 3 to 5 minutes.

Stir oil and chili butter into batter just until incorporated. Add vanilla and chocolate chips and blend just until incorporated. Batter will be thick and fudge-like.

To the Oven and Out
Spread batter evenly into prepared pan, smoothing top with a knife.

Place pan in preheated oven and bake for 24 to 28 minutes or until center is set. Let cool completely before slicing.

Each brownie contains 172 calories, 10g total fat, 4g saturated fat, 0g trans fat, 44mg cholesterol, 42mg sodium, 22g carbohydrate, 1g fiber, 2g protein.

*Allergy-friendly chocolate chips are available from Enjoy Life Foods (enjoylifefoods.com).

Lemon Sugar Cookies
Makes 36 cookies
(RECIPE BY MARY CAPONE)

Lemon extract makes these cookies burst with flavor. The dough holds up to any rolling pin, making these ideal for holiday cut-out cookies. This recipe can be made egg-free.*

Ingredients
1¼ cups Mary's All-Purpose Flour Blend
(page xiv)
½ cup tapioca starch/flour
½ cup potato starch (not potato flour)
2 teaspoons xanthan gum
1 teaspoon salt
1 cup unsalted butter or non-dairy
alternative, softened
1 cup sugar
1 large egg*
1 teaspoon pure vanilla extract
1 teaspoon gluten-free lemon extract

Getting Started

Lightly grease baking sheets or line them with parchment paper.

Making the Dough

In a large bowl, combine flour blend, tapioca starch/flour, potato starch, xanthan gum and salt. Set aside.

In the large bowl of a mixer, combine butter and sugar. Beat for 3 minutes until mixture is a pale yellow. Add in egg, vanilla extract and lemon extract.

Add dry ingredients, slowly mixing until dough forms. Place bowl in the refrigerator for 30 minutes.

Rolling Out Dough and Cutting Out Cookies

Preheat oven to 350°F. Remove half the dough and roll out onto a lightly floured surface to ¼-inch thickness. Use star shapes or other cookie cutters to cut out cookies and place them on prepared cookie sheets. Reroll scraps of dough. If dough becomes too sticky, chill again. Repeat with second half of dough.

To the Oven and Out

Bake in preheated oven 12 to 15 minutes until light brown. Remove and let cool thoroughly before handling and decorating.

> *For **Egg-Free Sugar Cookies,** omit 1 egg. Combine 1 tablespoon flax meal with 3 tablespoons hot water. Let sit 5 minutes until thickened. Add to recipe in place of 1 egg.

Royal Icing

1½ cups confectioners' sugar
1 large pasteurized egg white* or powdered egg white mixed with water to equal 1 egg white

½ teaspoon lemon juice
½ teaspoon gluten-free lemon extract
Food coloring

Making the Icing

Beat sugar and egg white with electric beater. Add lemon juice and lemon extract and beat until ingredients are incorporated.

Separate icing into small bowls and stir in a drop or 2 of different food coloring, as desired.

Chill icing until you're ready to decorate cooled cookies. Spread icing on cookies, as desired.

Each cookie with icing contains 125 calories, 5g total fat, 3g saturated fat, 0g trans fat, 19mg cholesterol, 79mg sodium, 19g carbo-hydrate, 0g fiber, 1g protein.

> *For **Egg-Free Royal Icing,** replace 1 egg white with 1½ teaspoons egg replacer mixed with 4 teaspoons warm water. Add mixture to sugar and proceed with recipe, as instructed. Gluten-free egg replacer is available from Ener-G Foods, (ener-g.com).

Key Lime Squares

Makes 24 squares
(RECIPE BY SUESON VESS)

This sweet-tart dessert is a great finish to a summertime picnic. It's also delicious when made with lemon juice. To store, pack squares in a tightly covered plastic container and refrigerate. This recipe can be made egg-free.*

Filling

Water
⅓ cup key lime juice, bottled or fresh squeezed
2 large egg yolks*
⅔ cup sugar
¼ cup cornstarch or arrowroot powder
Zest of 1 lime

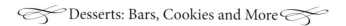

Crumb Mixture
1 cup *Living Without's* All-Purpose Flour Blend
(page xiv)
½ cup potato starch or cornstarch
1 teaspoon baking powder
1 teaspoon xanthan gum
½ teaspoon salt
½ cup + 3 tablespoons butter, non-dairy
alternative, or shortening
1 cup lightly packed brown sugar
1 cup quinoa flakes or gluten-free oats
Confectioners' sugar, optional

Getting Started
Preheat oven to 350°F. Line a 9x12-inch pan with foil. Grease the foil.

Making the Filling
To make filling, add enough water to lime juice to equal 1½ cups liquid. Whisk juice together with egg yolks, sugar, cornstarch and zest in a heavy-bottom saucepan and cook over low heat, stirring constantly until mixture has thickened and there are no lumps. Set aside to cool slightly.

Making the Squares
In a separate bowl, sift together flour blend, potato starch, baking powder, xanthan gum and salt. Set aside.

In a large bowl, cream butter or shortening. Add brown sugar and mix well.

Slowly add flour mixture to sugar mixture, scraping bowl often. Do not over-mix. Mixture will be crumbly. Stir quinoa flakes or oats.

To the Oven and Out
Firmly pat about half of the crumb mixture into the bottom of the prepared pan with your fingertips, making a smooth layer. Spoon the key lime filling over the crumb layer. Sprinkle remaining crumbs over the top of the filling. Some filling will show through.

Bake 30 to 35 minutes in preheated oven until lightly browned. Cool completely before cutting into squares. Sprinkle with confectioners' sugar before serving.

Each square contains 137 calories, 6g total fat, 3g saturated fat, 0g trans fat, 31g cholesterol, 79mg sodium, 21 total carbohydrates, 1g protein

> For **Egg-Free Key Lime Squares**, omit 2 egg yolks. Add 6 tablespoons unsweetened applesauce to lime juice before adding enough water to equal 1½ cups liquid as called for in the recipe. Add 1 extra tablespoon of cornstarch to filling. Bake an additional 10 to 15 minutes until the filling is firm. Cover if neccesary to prevent the crust from browning too quickly.

This recipe is reprinted with permission from *Simple, Delicious Solutions for Gluten-Free, Dairy-Free Cooking (Special Eats)*, by Sueson Vess.

S'mores Bars
Makes 24 bars
(RECIPE BY BETH HILLSON)

These bars have all the fixings of the popular campfire treat—chocolate, marshmallows and graham crackers. The campfire is optional. This recipe can be made egg-free.*

Ingredients
¾ cup (1½ sticks) unsalted butter or non-dairy
alternative, softened
1¼ cups sugar
2 large eggs*
2 teaspoons pure vanilla extract
2 cups *Living Without's* All-Purpose Flour
Blend (page xiv)
1½ cups gluten-free graham cracker crumbs

2 teaspoons baking powder
1½ teaspoons xanthan gum
¼ teaspoon salt
1½ cups chocolate chips
4 cups mini marshmallows

Getting Started

Preheat oven to 350°F. Line a 9x13-inch baking pan with foil, leaving a 2- to 3-inch overhang on 2 opposite ends.

Spray foil with vegetable oil.

Making the Dough

Beat butter and sugar in a large bowl until light and creamy. Add eggs and vanilla. Beat well.

In separate bowl, mix together flour, graham cracker crumbs, baking powder, xanthan gum and salt.

Add to butter mixture, beating until blended.

Putting It Together

Press half the dough into prepared pan. Sprinkle chocolate chips over dough. Sprinkle with marshmallows.

Scatter bits of remaining dough over marshmallows, pressing to cover the marshmallows. Don't worry if some marshmallows are showing.

To the Oven and Out

Place in preheated oven and bake 25 to 30 minutes or until lightly browned. Cool completely in pan on wire rack.

Lift out of pan by aluminum foil handles. Set on a smooth surface and cut into bars.

Each bar contains 256 calories,11g total fat, 6g saturated fat, 0g trans fat, 33mg cholesterol, 125mg sodium, 38g carbohydrate, 1g fiber, 2g protein.

*For **Egg-Free S'mores Bars,** omit 2 eggs. Add 1 tablespoon arrowroot to dry ingredients. Mix 2 tablespoons flax meal with 6 tablespoons warm water; let sit 5 minutes until slightly thickened. Add flax meal mixture to recipe to replace 2 eggs.

Substitution Solutions

DAIRY

Milk Replace 1 cup cow's milk with one of the following:

- 1 cup soy milk (plain)
- 1 cup rice milk
- 1 cup fruit juice
- 1 cup water
- 1 cup coconut milk
- 1 cup goat's milk, if tolerated
- 1 cup hemp milk

Buttermilk Replace 1 cup buttermilk with one of the following:

- 1 cup soy milk + 1 tablespoon lemon juice or 1 tablespoon cider vinegar (Let stand until slightly thickened.)
- 1 cup coconut milk
- 7/8 cup rice milk
- 7/8 cup fruit juice
- 7/8 cup water

Yogurt Replace 1 cup yogurt with one of the following:

- 1 cup soy yogurt or coconut yogurt
- 1 cup soy sour cream
- 1 cup unsweetened applesauce
- 1 cup fruit puree

Butter (1 stick = 8 tablespoons = ½ cup = 4 ounces) Replace 8 tablespoons butter with one of the following:

- 8 tablespoons Fleischmann's unsalted margarine;
- 8 tablespoons Earth Balance (Non-Dairy) Buttery Spread or Sticks;
- 8 tablespoons Spectrum Organic Shortening;
- 8 tablespoons vegetable or olive oil

For reduced fat:

- 6 tablespoons unsweetened applesauce + 2 tablespoons fat of choice

EGGS

Replace 1 large egg with one of the following:

Flax Gel: 1 tablespoon flax meal, chia seed or salba seed + 3 tablespoons hot water. (Let stand, stirring occasionally, about 10 minutes or until thickened. Use without straining.)

Egg Replacer: Egg Replacer, according to package directions

Tofu: 4 tablespoons pureed silken tofu + 1 teaspoon baking powder

Applesauce: 4 tablespoons unsweetened applesauce (or other fruit puree) + 1 teaspoon baking powder

IMPORTANT! Replacing more than two eggs will change the integrity of a recipe. For recipes that call for a lot of eggs, like a quiche, use pureed silken tofu. Because egg substitutions add moisture, you may have to increase baking times slightly.

Note: To replace one egg white, dissolve 1 tablespoon plain agar powder into 1 tablespoon water. Beat, chill for 15 minutes and beat again.

NUTS

Replace tree nuts or peanuts with an equal amount of one of the following:

Toasted coconut
Sunflower seeds
Toasted sesame seeds (use only 2 to 3 tablespoons)
Crushed gluten-free cornflakes
Crushed gluten-free crispy rice cereal
Crushed potato chips
Pumpkin seeds

Substitution Solutions

GLUTEN-FREE FLOUR

To make a flour blend, thoroughly combine all ingredients. Store in a covered container in the refrigerator until used. You can double or triple these recipes to make as much flour blend as you need. See pages xiii and xiv for additional flour blends used in this book.

Living Without's All-Purpose Flour Blend
MAKES 4 CUPS

Use this blend for most of your gluten-free baking.

- 2 cups rice flour (a combination of white and brown rice flour works well)
- 1 cup tapioca starch/flour
- 1 cup cornstarch or potato starch (not potato flour)

Each cup contains 436 calories, 1g total fat, 0g saturated fat, 0g trans fat, 0mg cholesterol, 99g carbohydrate, 3mg sodium, 2g fiber, 5g protein.

Living Without's High-Protein Flour Blend
MAKES 4½ CUPS

This nutritious blend works best in baked goods that require elasticity, such as wraps and pie crusts.

- 1¼ cups bean flour (of choice), chickpea flour or soy flour
- 1 cup white or brown rice flour
- 1 cup arrowroot starch, cornstarch or potato starch (not potato flour)
- 1 cup tapioca starch/flour

Each cup contains 588 calories, 3g total fat, 0g saturated fat, 0g trans fat, 0mg cholesterol, 128g carbohydrate, 24mg sodium, 6g fiber, 11g protein.

General Guidelines for Using Xanthan or Guar Gum

Gum (xanthan or guar) is the key to successful gluten-free baking. It provides the binding needed to give the baked product proper elasticity, keeping it from crumbling.

- Add ½ teaspoon xanthan or guar gum per cup of flour blend to make cakes, cookies, bars, muffins and other quick breads.

- Add 1 teaspoon per cup of flour blend to make yeast bread, pizza dough or other baked items that call for yeast.

Note: If you purchase a commercial flour blend, read the ingredient list carefully. Some blends contain salt and xanthan or guar gum. If so, there is no need to add more.

Nutritional analyses of recipes in this book are based on data supplied by the U.S. Department of Agriculture and certain food companies. Nutrient amounts are approximate due to variances in product brands, manufacturing and actual preparation.

Shopping List

For gluten-free or allergy-friendly ingredients, check out these resources.

Adobo Seasoning
Goya Foods
goya.com

Penzeys Spices
penzeys.com

Spicely Organic Spices
spicely.com

The Spice House
thespicehouse.com

Bread Crumbs
Bob's Red Mill
bobsredmill.com

Gillian's Foods
gilliansfoodsglutenfree.com

Glutino
glutino.com

Broth
College Inn
collegeinn.com

Imagine Foods
imaginefoods.com

Pacific Foods
pacificfoods.com

Shelton's
sheltons.com

Swanson
swansonbroth.com

Butter Alternatives
Earth Balance
earthbalancenatural.com

Spectrum
spectrumorganics.com

Canned Pumpkin
Farmer's Market Foods
farmersmarketfoods.com

Pacific Foods
pacificfoods.com

Cheese (dairy-free)
Daiya Foods
daiyafoods.com

Follow Your Heart
followyourheart.com

Go Veggie!
goveggiefoods.com

Lisanatti Foods
lisanattifoods.com

Tofutti
tofutti.com

Chocolate Chips
Enjoy Life Foods
enjoylifefoods.com

Cream Cheese
Follow Your Heart
followyourheart.com

GO Veggie!
goveggiefoods.com

Egg Replacer
Ener-G Foods
ener-g.com

Flour Blends
1-2-3 Gluten Free
123glutenfree.com

Kinnikinnick Foods
kinnikinnick.com

Mina's Purely Divine
minasgf.com

Tom Sawyer
glutenfreeflour.com

Flour Blends (whole grain)
Authentic Foods
authenticfoods.com

Bob's Red Mill
bobsredmill.com

King Arthur Flour
kingarthurflour.com

Flour (specialty)
Koda Farms
kodafarms.com

Lundberg Family Farms
lundberg.com

Premium Gold
premiumgoldflax.com

Food Coloring
Durkee
durkee.com

India Tree
indiatree.com

McCormick
mccormick.com

Shopping List

Food Coloring
continued

Nature's Flavors
naturesflavors.com

Seelect Tea
seelecttea.com

Spice Islands
spiceislands.com

Mayonnaise
Mindful Mayo
earthbalancenatural.com

Nasoya
nasoya.com

Organicville
organicvillefoods.com

Spectrum
spectrumorganics.com

Vegenaise
followyourheart.com

Oats (gluten-free)
Bob's Red Mill
bobsredmill.com

Cream Hill Estates
creamhillestates.com

Gifts of Nature
giftsofnature.net

Gluten Free Oats
glutenfreeoats.com

Glutenfreeda Foods
glutenfreedafoods.com

Pepperoni
Applegate Farms
applegate.com

Dietz & Watson
dietzandwatson.com

Hormel Foods
hormelfoods.com

Wellshire Farms
wellshirefarms.com

Pie Crust Mix
Authentic Foods
authenticfoods.com

Gluten-Free Pantry
glutino.com

Moon Rabbit Foods
moonrabbitfoods.com

Williams-Sonoma
williams-sonoma.com

Pizza Sauce
Eden Foods
edenfoods.com

Muir Glen
muirglen.com

Powdered Milk
Better Than Milk (rice, soy)
btmsoymilk.com

Meyenberg Goat Milk Products (goat milk)
meyenberg.com

Nature's Flavors (soy)
naturesflavors.com

Vance's Foods (potato)
vancesfoods.com

Sausage
Aidells Sausage Company
aidells.com

Al Fresco
alfrescoallnatural.com

Applegate Farms
applegate.com

Beeler's
beelerspurepork.com

Coleman Natural
colemannatural.com

Jones Dairy Farm
jonesdairyfarm.com

Shortening
(organic, non-hydrogenated)
Earth Balance
earthbalancenatural.com

Spectrum
spectrumorganics.com

Sour Cream
Follow Your Heart
followyourheart.com

Tofutti
tofutti.com

Tortillas, Wraps
Food for Life
foodforlife.com

French Meadow Bakery
frenchmeadow.com

La Tortilla Factory
latortillafactory.com

Whipped Topping
MimicCreme
mimiccreme.com

Shopping List

Yogurt
Chobani
chobani.com

Fage
fageusa.com

Green Valley Organics
greenvalleylactosefree.com

So Delicious
sodeliciousdairyfree.com

Not every product sold by every company listed is gluten-free or allergy-friendly. Read labels carefully. When in doubt, confirm ingredients directly with the manufacturer.

Index

Index

Index

Index

Index

Index

Index

Index

Index